Dr. Sebi Herbs and Food l

How to Naturally Heal and Revitalize your Body through Dr. Sebi Nutritional Guide with Effective Herbal Antibiotics to stay Healthy and begins to weight loss since day 1

By

Oliver Hendry

Dr. Sebi Diet

Table of Contents

Introduction

Diet by Dr. Sebi has been very popular but it has several drawbacks along with the advantages. It detoxify or cleanse the body from toxins and helps the body organs function efficiently. This diet mainly focuses on the plant based food and requires to skip completely synthetic, processed, GMF and other seedless fruits. This will help to lose weight, remove toxins from the body and keeping the body healthy. However, it is not budget friendly to follow this diet and it may lead to several nutrient deficiencies as it does not allow to consume meat and meat products, dairy and dairy products, limits the fruit choices and herbs etc. Liver and kidneys are the main organs that help the body to naturally detoxify the body and this diet will help to improve the function of these organs. This diet gives these organs relaxation from their work. Food items and herbs that are allowed to be consume are documented. There are also natural ways to detoxify the body. Choosing healthy and organic food with healthy lifestyle will help to achieve the optimal health status. Even if it restricts many food items, still it can help make variety of dishes and you can enjoy that as well.

Chapter 1: Dr. Sebi

In this chapter, you will learn about the founder of this diet and will make you familiar with what the diet actually is. Although diet by Dr. Sebi lacks scientific approaches it still has many health benefits. These health benefits are to help preventing the serious health conditions such as diabetes, heart disease, liver disease, and kidney or stomach disorders. Other than disease preventions, it helps to improve the immunity, makes you feel energized and more focused on your day to day tasks. It will also help you to lose weight. It is difficult to stick to the certain diet for a longer period of time, so for that few tips are also mentioned in this chapter to help you stay motivated and stick to this diet.

1.1 Alfredo Bowman

There are a lot of options for dieting to lose weight, from recent diet shows and Instagram influencers venting their current dream food pill. And with lots of contradictory facts on which one is better, it's hard to distinguish reality from myth, except though someone who appears credible suggests a diet.

Take the Diet by Dr. Sebi, the second in most-search Internet diet for 2019, for example. While others believe that a physician named Alfredo Bowman developed the program, and is the creator, was not a physician but an herbalist.

While it insists on consuming vegetarian diet and avoiding refined products that may be helpful, diet by Dr. Sebi is often highly stringent and lacks nutrients and protein. Prior to thinking of following diet by Dr. Sebi, here's what you should get to know:

Who was He?

Dr. Sebi whose real name was Alfredo Bowman, was a Honduran-born, self-taught herbalist. He had been educated on his own and did not have specific medical experience, according to his biography. He wasn't a practitioner, neither did he possess a Ph.D.

He settled in America and was cared unsuccessfully for his multiple medical illnesses, plus asthma, diabetes, impotence, and obesity. It is said that Bowman was cured in Mexico with the help of an herbalist who encouraged him to make herbal combinations on his own, which he named Cell Food by Dr. Sebi.

He initially claimed that these combinations of herbs can treat medical diseases like HIV, sickle cell anaemia, and lupus. Nevertheless, he was charged in 1987 (although the jury convicted him) for working as medicine expert without a permit. After an additional litigation by the New York State a few years back, Sebi promised to avoid making promises that his drugs could treat any ailments.

Though debated, Sebi has reportedly received a number of clients: Michael Jackson, Steven Seagal, and John Travolta.

Sebi was detained in 2016 for currency exempting. He developed pneumonia whilst incarcerated in Honduras, and collapsed on his way to the hospital.

What is the diet by Dr. Sebi?

He believed that the illness is a consequence of acidity and mucus in the bloodstream, and concluded that in a high pH atmosphere infections could not occur. His plan, which requires a rather stringent nutritional regime and costly vitamins, claims to detoxify the disease body and preserve alkalinity (no clinical evidence is sufficient to back up his statements).

The lifestyle excludes every sort of animal food and generally relies on vegetarian diet but with even more rigorous guidelines. This excludes seedless fruits, for example, and only allows Sebi's authorized list of "organic growing foods."

Is Diet by Dr. Sebi healthy?

This diet is extremely protein deficient: Sebi does not approve any food from animal origin, eggs, milk, and soy as well. He also restrains certain legumes and beans. Some "naturally grown grains," walnuts, Brazil nuts, and hemp seeds are the only items to provide some protein in the diet. This may be very challenging to satisfy dietary requirements from certain products alone.

A significant component of any cell of the body, is protein and the nutrition the body uses to help regenerate develop and tissues. It is also an important bone, skin, tissue, cartilage and blood building component. Restricting the main macronutrients and food groups will contribute to deficits in nutrition and malnutrition.

Although it encourages certain vegetables and fruits, it strangely limits the number of items. It calls for plum or cherry tomatoes for starters and nothing else from it. Certain types he excludes are mushrooms (shiitake) and lettuce (Iceberg) which allows the diet much more stringent, rendering follow-up very challenging.

Sebi's key focus is on the supplements made by him, which make ambitious claims that they will "accelerate the healing cycle" and "rejuvenate and participate in intercellular advancement." Many packets cost up to 1500 dollars and do not mention any nutrient or quantity specifics. It makes it impossible to learn the quantity of nutrients you receive from his patented mixtures and what precisely is in his products.

Beyond everything, He is in no form or shape a practitioner and there is no scientific research to back up his arguments and recommendations. The extremely restraining dietary recommendations promote the removal of macronutrients and major food groups that can negatively affect your health, which, not to mention, can lead to a toxic relationship with diet. Knowing the truth and knowing your science confirms whatever plan you adopt is important not to slip into a diet conspiracy trap.

1.2 Benefits of the Diet by Dr Sebi

Diet by Dr. Sebi is very low in fat, saturated fats and refined products, plus it does not include cholesterol, added sugar or alcohol. Many people lose weight as they eat this way, and because of the lack of meat products, processed goods, and carbohydrates, there is a significant decrease in the likelihood of some diseases correlated with their consumption:

- Cardiac attack

- Higher blood pressure

- Type 2 diabetes

- Stroke

- Cancer

- High cholesterol

As in most vegan programs, diet by Dr. Sebi calls for supplementation especially vitamin B-12. Calcium, iron, and omega-3 fatty acids may also be added, but most of such important nutrients can be derived from whole food plant-based foods altogether. If you don't get ample access to sunshine, you'll probably want vitamin D supplementation.

Reducing the intake of acidic food results in lowering the production of mucus in the body, and produce an alkaline atmosphere that makes illness quite difficult to develop. It's much easier to use herbs in your approach to cleansing your body.

Weight Loss with Diet by Dr. Sebi

Each segment is straight forward. To lose weight is expected to occur following a diet because the diet by Dr. Sebi comprises of raw foods, grains, fruits, legumes, and nuts.

This cuts down waste, milk, processed food and meat, and you'll lose weight, obviously. Diet by Dr. Sebi works as a detox or cleanse and is reaping other rewards including gratitude to the body.

Strengthens Immunity

Illnesses and diseases derive from a poor immune system. Many say to have improved their immunity and to have been recovered from other illnesses by faithfully practicing the diet by Dr. Sebi and everyone knows that medication does not heal ailments.

Reduced Risk of Disease

Food items that are of acidic nature corrode the slimy layer of the body's cells and internal linings, contributing to a weakened system that renders disease possibility and a treatment unthinkable. Consequently, consuming alkaline diets will reduce the likelihood of disease and help the body get what it wants to nourish the cells that are productive.

Reduction in Hypertension and Stroke Risk

First-line treatments for all levels of hypertension require fitness and weight reduction, according to the National Institute of Health (NIH). However, the findings of one limited cross-sectional analysis show that the more significant therapy is a vegetarian diet than medication and regular medicinal method itself.

The advantages of a vegetarian diet relative to medication, noting that a vegetarian diet could reduce fat deposition in the blood vessels, and decrease the possibility of heart disease stroke, and diabetes, in the medical studies they examined.

The alkaline electric diet by Dr Sebi is a modified variant of a vegan diet focused on plants.

Energy

Diets that are high in meat, milk and processed crystal sugar may be a drain on levels of energy of the body. Focusing on vegetarian diet for living is a healthier way, as it will improve the vitality you regularly exhibit.

Increased Focus

Ensuing the teachings of Dr Sebi would help remove the cloud of the brain, keep you centered and less distracted by the unpleasant circumstances that happen.

Also if you're not sick, following an approach focused on plants will benefit you in leading a good, safe life.

Dr. Sebi Diet

1.3 Guidelines for Following the Diet for Long-term

This one can require time and commitment like every other diet you're working to achieve! Although it can be demanding at first, the body should gradually get accustomed to the novel form of eating. When you remove all the unhealthy things you might have eaten previously in your life, you may continue to feel more energized. There are some of the tips and instructions to adopt to make this journey the most fun and enjoyable.

Drink Lots of Water

Individuals must be consuming at least 4-5 liters of water a day according to Bowman. This is important to make the diet by Dr. Sebi function at its best of capacity. Alfredo prefers fresh spring water from a reverse osmosis device, as opposed to water obtained through any other procedure. Several organizations working for human health and nutrition experts are often recommending 4-5 liters of water a day. Remember that water extracts waste products out of the body thereby aiding in nutrient digestion and cushioning of organs and joints.

Emotional and Mental Preparedness for the Diet

This would be very probable that you have developed certain deep patterns consuming those sorts of foodstuffs every day that may find it really challenging to quit or modify your food. Your friends and family can even pose a barrier while attempting to adopt the diet of Dr Sebi. Before you start this program, try to focus on thinking that why you want to improve your diet and the emotional and mental challenges that you probably will encounter.

Don't Quit Snacking

Yeah, you did understand correctly! Though you don't have to quit on the snacking, the best way to snack is eat healthy. That means consuming a slice of fruit or making treats focused on the suggested food plan, instead of opting for a packet of processed chips.

Analyze the Permitted Foods

Dr. Sebi Diet

Try your utmost not to depart from the authorized food list as this can delay your output. Although eating from the chosen list can seem too hard at first, you will soon find it easier than you expected particularly if you're mentally prepared.

Incorporate Whole Foods in Your Daily Diet

Make any attempt to periodically substitute processed products with whole products in your daily diet. You want to dodge processed foods because they are loaded with additives which can be very compelling, particularly when many have refined carbohydrates which triggers cravings in food.

Cooking Food is Compulsory

You can soon notice that the diet by Dr Sebi needs to be cooked as you begin. The guides provide food recipes which are not acidic to encourage this method. His guides take you through an alkaline meal, step by step. When you start cooking food for yourself, you can see that you can make your own favorite dishes with accepted ingredients and cook them with it.

1.4 Why You Should Pass on diet by Dr. Sebi?

1. It's Misleading

Unlike several many fad diets (GM diet), the diet by Dr. Sebi doesn't have any clear evidence to back the arguments. Not only does the diet rely on company-sold products, but also the name is deceptive because Dr. Sebi (whose real name is Alfredo Bowman) may not currently have any certificates or certifications.

His reputation gives the diet more legitimacy, which making you believe it's a reliable diet because he's not even a doctor at all. "One point is that you just ought to be wary about every plan if anyone markets things to you, or vitamins, rather than providing advice about what to do." Moreover, the promises of the plan to detoxify and heal the body are deceptive and actually dangerous. Your kidneys and liver are still very successful at eliminating contaminants from the body, so there is little proof that it will either improve or inhibit this cycle with other products or supplements.

Dr. Sebi Diet

2. It May Lead to Nutrient Deficiencies

The diet by Dr. Sebi would definitely leave you short when it comes to your nutrition, particularly where protein is concerned. While the diet requires nuts and seeds with certain protein content, the total absence of certain animal products would possibly leave you lacking in protein.

Although your protein requirements can be fulfilled on a plant-based diet, doing so may be difficult. And the prohibition of unhealthy products in the diet Dr. Sebi (such as tofu or veggie burgers, for example) and vitamins outside the diet's own drug will make things much tougher (if not impossible) to get what your body requires.

the average individual requires approximately 7 grams of protein per 20 pounds of body weight per day. So if you weigh 160 pounds a day, you will eat around 56 grams of protein. For the background, according to USDA's FoodData Central, a 1-ounce serving of Sebi-approved walnuts provides just over 4 grams of protein.

Restricting animal products can often leave you deprived of omega-3 fatty acids. Omega-3s are important for general brain activity and contribute to memory and efficiency. Deficiency, among others, may contribute to symptoms such as exhaustion, impaired memory, dry skin, and heart disease.

3. It is Unsustainable

In addition, diet by Dr. Sebi discourages all refined foods, which is not inherently healthy. Ultra-packaged products usually do not offer significant health benefits (think: chips and cookies), but packaged items such as preserved fruits or vegetables may be part of a safe, nutritious diet. Not only are they nutritious, easily accessible, and easy to prepare with — making meal cooking even more doable — but many of these packaged products are often packed with nutrients that the typical consumer would not be able to get through their normal eating habits.

On the other side, Dr. Sebi-approved products can be difficult to get by in the regular store or diner, and tougher to cook at home, rendering the diet pretty challenging to stick within the long term.

The Bottom Line

Although the focus of diet of Dr. Sebi is on consuming lots of vegetables and fruit that is certainly a good feature of another faulty diet, this is not a plan that can offer several advantages. You should Include more whole foods into your diet is not a terrible thing either, but the extremely stringent aspect of this approach makes it impossible to provide the range of nutrients that your body requires.

Particularly for those following the diet by Dr. Sebi as a way of treating or alleviating an illness or injury, prioritizing a health care professional's advice is important. Before you try this sort of diet, it is better to speak to the doctor and make sure it's a good option for you.

Chapter 2: Detoxification and Cleansing

This chapter will give you a complete insight about what is detoxification and cleansing and what is the difference between them and in what context they are used interchangeably. There are more than one approaches to detoxify the body. Basic steps towards cleansing or detoxification are also discussed in detail for example limit alcohol, be physically active, get enough and sound sleep, consume fresh and organic food items, try to avoid processed food items. According to the results required, there are different types of detox diets that are being used for example weight loss etc. Few of the major disadvantages of detoxification are dehydration, deficiency of certain nutrient and digestive problems.

2.1 When and How to do it?

A number of foods, regimens, and treatments for "detoxification "— sometimes labelled" detoxes "or" cleanses "— have been proposed as methods to eliminate contaminants from the body, reduce weight or improve health.

The words cleanse, and detox are also used interchangeably, and although both extract contaminants from the body, they are two separate things detox and cleanse! The term "cleanse" means clean at the root, so you should think about a cleanse as a way of cleaning the body. A cleanse also utilizes supplements or medicines to specifically remove toxins and usually concentrates on the digestive tract. On the other side, detox methods aim to help the normal mechanisms for the removal of contaminants in the body. As the major detoxifying centers of the body are the liver and the kidneys, successful detox programs concentrate on helping the liver and kidneys and supplying them with the nutrients and vitamins they need to function optimally.

And what are toxins? Heavy metals like mercury are top of mind, but chronic chemical contaminants, plastics, and pesticides are still found on the list. Toxins are simply harmful contaminants that will remain in the system, irritate cells, induce inflammation, and interact with regular functions in the body.

Dr. Sebi Diet

Signs of toxicity or extreme toxicity (and hence the need for detoxification or cleansing) include:

- Exhaustion

- Headaches

- Joint pain

- Depression

- Anxiety

- Constipation

The Cleansing Journey

Cleansing is related to maintain the gut clean. The digestive system is the way through which the body absorbs its nutrients. When it becomes toxic, it is sluggish in performing its roles. A build-up of waste in the intestine may become harmful, resulting in pain and sickness. Bloating is one indication of an unstable gut. It is attributed to gas build-up because the body isn't getting rid of waste as it would. Then, the food starts to decompose. Nutrition is supposed to be sustainable and only as natural as nature. the digestive tract also includes helpful and hazardous microbes. If these bacteria's equilibrium is disrupted, so it contributes to problems. Purging is the most common method of cleaning where a laxative is used to eliminate fecal matter, bacteria, and all other unnecessary material. The trouble to follow this strategy, however, is that it's non-selective and clears the good along with the poor. This may also be harmful because, during the cycle, you may lose enough water, which would make you dehydrated. Another way the body gets rid of toxic chemicals is by consuming lots of water. Exercise and adequate sleep are crucial to helping you succeed in the cleaning program.

A successful detox strategy is to carry out the cycle of curing the stomach and taking note of what goes through it. Fast food is so-called because it doesn't have the nutrition the body requires. Rather it threatens to mess up the intestinal tract by obstructing it. Foods, including wheat, soy, sugar, milk, and caffeine, can be removed and substituted

Dr. Sebi Diet

by organic replacements that have not been refined and contaminated. The cleansing cycle is not complete simply by removing the waste of the digestive tract. This needs to be treated by supplying nutritious food that can make the gut function at its fullest. This involves balanced food with adequate fiber and that which will help maintain safe environment levels, including good bacteria in the intestine. Organic beverages such as unflavored probiotic yogurt often help.

To continue the cleaning system, you need to go through a pre-cleanse process where you need to cut back on alcohol and numerous unhealthy foods. However, when the body started adapting and starting to work properly, it is realized that energy thresholds are far stronger.

The Detox Route

Detox is another method of removing harmful chemicals from the body. The body usually gets rid of contaminants through the skin, liver, and kidneys. Detox would strengthen the work of certain organs. So, what contaminants are the cycle aiming for? For one aspect, the air you inhale is full of chemicals that make their way through your body, where they lodge and create discomfort. Some foods, too, contain contaminants such as toxins, preservatives, and tastes. In this time period, meat should be avoided.

Your skin is often loaded with a mixture of chemicals contained in the lotions, creams, and other products that you use. Occasionally, the organs associated with detoxification are overloaded. Foods such as lemon, garlic, kale, pineapple, and ginger can help detoxify the body. You can speak to a nutritionist about these, because others may have harmful consequences. Garlic, for instance, thins the blood, which could threaten someone whose blood doesn't readily clot. Food supplements, too, help enhance the functionality of the kidneys and liver.

2.2 What are some detoxification/Cleansing approaches?

In an integrative health-care model, several detoxification therapies are provided.

• Exercise/movement

Dr. Sebi Diet

- Body-mind relaxation (yoga, exercise, mindfulness, prayer)

- Pure/alkaline water

- Diet

- Fasting

- Juicing

- Supplements

- Detox treatment and body scrubs

- Infrared sauna

- Lymphatic drainage

- Ozonetherapy (autohemotherapy)

- Detox infusions

- Colon hydrotherapy

- Osteopathy

2.3 Why Detoxification/Cleansing?

In essence, there are eight forms in which toxins destroy our bodies, which need detoxification.

Toxins poison enzymes so they do not function effectively.

Our bodies are the engines of the enzymes. Every physiological process relies on enzymes to produce molecules, generate energy, and build cellular structures. Toxins disrupt enzymes and thus weaken myriad body functions — inhibiting, for example, the development of hemoglobin in the blood, or reducing the body's ability to resist free-radical disruption that accelerates aging.

Toxins result in weaker bones by displacing structural minerals.

For lifetime mobility, people must preserve stable bone mass. There is a twofold consequence as toxins displace the calcium contained throughout the bone: weakened skeletal systems and increased toxins emitted through bone degradation, which spread across the body.

Toxins damage the organs.

Toxins destroy virtually any organ and cell that you have. When the digestive system, liver, and kidneys are so acidic that they cannot detoxify efficiently, then your detoxification will backfire, and the body will stay acidic.

Toxins increase the rate of aging and degeneration by damaging the DNA.

Many widely used pesticides, phthalates, poorly detoxified estrogens, and benzene drugs are DNA-damaging.

Toxins modify gene expression.

Our genes are always switching off and on to respond to shifts in our bodies and the conditions outside. But there are many toxins that trigger or suppress our genes in unwanted ways.

Toxins make cell membranes to do not respond effectively.

"Signaling" exists in the cell membranes inside the body. Harm to these membranes prevents them from obtaining essential messages — insulin that does not, for example, warn the cells to absorb more sugar, or muscle cells that do not react to signal from magnesium to relax.

Toxins interfere with hormones and cause imbalances.

Toxins are chemicals that stimulate, suppress, imitate, and obstruct. One example: Arsenic disrupts the receptors of thyroid hormones in the cells, such that the cells do not obtain the message from the thyroid hormones that allow them to revive metabolism. The effect is unexplained fatigue.

Last but not least, contaminants potentially hinder the detoxification ability — and this is the worst of all.

It is easier to achieve when you are very acidic and really need to detoxify than when you are not acidic. In other words, even as you really need your detox schemes (to fix health problems), your hard-working detox scheme would more definitely perform below average. Why? For what? Because you're already bearing strong toxic load has exceeded your detox potential. That's Right. The more toxic compounds you have built up in your body, the greater the damage to your body's detoxification pathways.

That's why sustaining your detox organs — and your detox systems with them — is such an essential undertaking. The end effect is you will instead remove contaminants quickly from the body.

Conclusion

If you still suffer from bowel irritation, consider cleansing. When you are exhausted and suffer from fatigue, insomnia, and anxiety, the need for detox is typically suggested. You should adopt a system of cleansing because it has long-term, even life-long effects. Typically, detox is a short-term procedure that restores the body to control after contaminants have built up.

2.4 Misconceptions about Detoxing

Detox diets are known to remove the body's contaminants, boost overall health, and facilitate loss of weight. They also require the use of laxatives, teas, vitamins, diuretics, minerals and products, which are believed to be detoxifying. The word "toxin" is poorly described in the sense of these diets. Typically it contains pollutants, synthetic products, refined foods and heavy metals — all of which have a detrimental health impact. Common detox diets seldom, however, describe the actual contaminants that they focus to extract or the process by which they ostensibly eradicate.

Moreover, there is little data to justify the usage of such diets for removing contaminants or for weight loss. Your body uses complex method to remove contaminants affecting the liver, digestive tract, lungs and skin. Even, they will only successfully remove harmful contaminants while certain parts are healthy. And while

Dr. Sebi Diet

these diets do nothing your body actually cannot do things on its own, however, you can maximize the normal detoxification mechanism in your body.

2.5 Steps towards Detoxification/Cleansing

1. Focus on Sleep

Ensuring adequate and regular quality sleep is a must for supporting the health and natural detoxification system of your body. Sleeping allows the brain to reorganize and refresh itself, to eliminate by-products and hazardous contaminants that have accrued all day long. One of the waste products is a protein known as beta-amyloid, which contributes to Alzheimer's disease progression. Your body does not have time to conduct certain tasks with sleeplessness, and contaminants will build up and influence many health facets.

Short- and long-term health effects such as tension, anxiety, elevated blood pressure, heart disease, type 2 diabetes, and obesity have been linked with inadequate sleep. You should usually sleep 7 to 9 hours a night to promote better health. If you are facing trouble with falling asleep or staying asleep at night, behavioral changes such as sticking to a sleep routine and reducing blue light — produced by mobile devices and computer screens — are helpful in optimizing sleep prior to bed. Adequate sleep helps the brain to reorganize, regenerate, and eliminate contaminants that build all day long.

2. Limit Alcohol

About 90 percent of the alcohol is processed by the liver. Enzymes of liver metabolizes the alcohol into the familiar cancer producing compounds acetaldehyde. When acetaldehyde is known as a poison, the liver transforms it into a harmless product named acetate that is then excreted out of the body.

While clinical trials have found that moderate to low alcohol intake is safe for health of heart, alcoholism can trigger a variety of health problems. By inducing accumulation of fat, scarring, and inflammation, heavy drinking can seriously impair your liver function. If that occurs, the liver can't work properly and conduct the necessary

Dr. Sebi Diet

functions — like removing the body's waste and other chemicals. Limiting or fully abstaining from alcohol as such is few of the easiest ways to maintain the body's system of detoxication run smoothly. Health officials are proposing that alcohol consumption should be limited to one drink a day for women and 2 for men. If you don't drink at all, you shouldn't start for the possibility of benefits of hearts associated with moderate to mild drinking. Drinking too much alcohol can reduce the capacity of the liver to conduct its usual processes, such as detoxification.

3. Drink More Water

Water has a lot more functions than just quenching the thirst. It controls your body temperature, lubricates joints, assists in digestion and absorption of nutrients, and detoxifies the body by eliminating wastes. The cells in your body will be restored constantly to work optimally and break down the nutrients that your body requires to use as energy. However, such processes produce waste — in the form of urea and carbon dioxide — which, if left to build up in your blood, will cause damage. Water carries these waste materials, efficiently eliminating them by urination, respiration, or sweating. So it is essential to remain properly hydrated for detoxification.

Sufficient regular water consumption for men is 125 ounces (3.7 liters), and for women is 91 ounces (2.7 liters). Depending on your health, where you stay, and the degree of exercise, you may require more or less. Water helps the body's detoxification mechanism to extract toxic materials from your blood, in addition to the other functions in the body.

4. Focus on Sleep

Ensuring adequate and regular quality sleep is a must for supporting the health and natural detoxification system of your body. Sleeping allows the brain to reorganize and refresh itself, to eliminate by-products and hazardous contaminants that have accrued all day long. One of the waste products is a protein known as beta-amyloid, which contributes to Alzheimer's disease progression. Your body does not have time to

Dr. Sebi Diet

conduct certain tasks with sleeplessness, and contaminants will build up and influence many health facets.

Short- and long-term health effects such as tension, anxiety, elevated blood pressure, heart disease, type 2 diabetes, and obesity have been linked with inadequate sleep. You should usually sleep 7 to 9 hours a night to promote better health. If you are facing trouble with falling asleep or staying asleep at night, behavioral changes such as sticking to a sleep routine and reducing blue light — produced by mobile devices and computer screens — are helpful in optimizing sleep prior to bed. Adequate sleep helps the brain to reorganize, regenerate, and eliminate contaminants that build all day long.

5. Eat foods rich with antioxidants

Antioxidants shield the cells from the harm that molecules known as free radicals can do. Oxidative stress is a situation induced by free radicals being generated too rapidly. Such molecules are normally generated by your body for cellular processes, for example, digestion. However, excessive free radicals may be created by alcohol, cigarette smoke, unhealthy diet, and exposure to pollutants. These compounds have been used in a variety of disorders, such as dementia, heart diseases, liver disease, different forms of cancer, asthma, by creating harm to the body's cells. Eating an antioxidant-rich diet can help your body tackle oxidative stress due to the excessive amount of other toxins and free radicals that increase the risk of illness. Focus on having antioxidants the food not the supplements, which, when taken in large amounts, can potentially increase the risk of certain diseases.

Copious research indicates whole foods like cruciferous plants, berries, garlic, and spices such as turmeric can help detoxify the body via specific pathways. Paired with protein and quality fat provides an ideal strategy for detoxifying and reducing the weight of the body. Whenever possible, opt for sustainable plant products and the best quality animal foods. These contain vitamin C, vitamin E, vitamin A, zeaxanthin, lutein, and selenium. Nuts, berries, fruits chocolate, vegetables, spices, and beverages such as coffee and green tea contain some of the very high levels of antioxidants. Having an

Dr. Sebi Diet

antioxidant-rich diet helps the body minimize the harm done by free radicals and can reduce the risk of diseases that may affect detoxification.

6. Decrease the Intake of Sugar and Processed Foods

Sugar and processed products are known to be at the center of the latest public health problems. High sugar and highly refined food intake are linked with obesity and other chronic diseases such as heart disease, cancer, and diabetes. These diseases hamper your body's ability to detoxify itself naturally by harming organs, such as your liver and kidneys that play an important role.

High intake of sugary drinks, for example, may induce fatty liver, a disease that has a detrimental impact on liver function. Through consuming less fast food, you will preserve safe detoxification function throughout your body. Leaving it on the store shelf can reduce junk food. Not seeing it in your kitchen takes away the opportunity. Often a good way of minimizing intake is to substitute processed food with nutritious alternatives like fruits and vegetables. An unhealthy intake of processed food is linked with chronic illnesses such as obesity and diabetes. Such disorders can damage organs such as the liver and kidneys, which are essential for detoxification.

7. Decrease the intake of salt

To others, detoxification is a way to remove excess water. A lot of salt may cause the body to absorb excess liquid, especially if you have a disease that affects your liver or kidneys — or if you do not drink enough water. The excess accumulation of fluid can cause bloating. If you catch yourself consuming too much salt, you will detoxify yourself from the excess water of the body.

Although it may feel counterintuitive, one of the easiest strategies to remove extra water weight by eating so much salt is by increasing your sodium consumption. Its how the body produces a hormone that is antidiuretic. It stops you from doing urine– and thereby detoxifying – when you consume so much salt and not enough water. By increasing the consumption of fluids, the body decreases antidiuretic hormone production, and improves urination, removing both water and waste materials.

Dr. Sebi Diet

Often tends to boost the consumption of products rich with potassium – which counterbalances some of the impacts of sodium. Foods rich with potassium include squash, potato, bananas, spinach and kidney beans. Taking too much salt will improve the retention of water. By increasing the consumption of water and foods rich with potassium, you will minimize extra water-and waste.

8. Eat Foods High in Prebiotics

Gastrointestinal disorders may produce a dysfunctional detoxification system, or worsen it. Improving the digestive system involves eliminating inhibitors that generate dysbiosis (good imbalances) and other issues while also adding the correct foods and nutrients to benefit the gut. If you fear intestinal permeability (leaky intestine), or any stomach issues, speak to the chiropractor or certain health-care practitioners. Gut health is significant in maintaining a healthy detoxification system. Your intestinal cells have a mechanism of detoxification and excretion that defends the gut and body from dangerous toxins, including chemicals. Good gut health begins with prebiotics, a type of fiber that feeds the good bacteria that are called probiotics in your gut. Your healthy bacteria will generate nutrients, called short-chain fatty acids, with prebiotics that are helpful for health. Because of antibiotic usage, inadequate oral hygiene, and food consistency, the healthy bacteria in your gut will become unbalanced with bad bacteria.

This unhealthy shift in bacteria can, therefore, weaken your immune and detoxification systems and increase your risk of illness and inflammation. Consuming prebiotic-rich foods will keep the immune systems and detoxification strong. Good prebiotic food sources include tomatoes, artichokes, bananas, asparaguses, onions, garlic, and oats. Eating a prebiotic-rich diet keeps your digestive system healthy, which is critical for proper detoxification and immune health.

9. Get Active

Regular activity — regardless of body weight — is correlated with a longer lifespan and decreased incidence of multiple illnesses and disorders, including type 2 diabetes, cardiac failure, elevated blood pressure, and some cancers. Although there are many

Dr. Sebi Diet

reasons behind exercise's health benefits, the main factor is reduced inflammation. While some inflammation is required to rebound from injury or repair wounds, too much of it weakens the structures in your body and causes disease. Exercise will help the body's processes – like the detoxification mechanism – work better and defend against illness by reducing inflammation. It's recommended that you do moderate-intensity exercise at least 150–300 minutes a week, such as brisk walking or vigorous-intensity physical activity such as running.

10. Reduce inflammation

Toxicity contributes to inflammation, which leads to a heavier toxic load, which in turn prevents fat loss in return. An anti-inflammatory diet contains wild seafood, omega-3-rich plant foods, including flaxseed and chia seeds, plenty of non-starchy vegetables, and spices, including turmeric. Check with the chiropractor or other health care providers to add anti-inflammatory foods into your diet, including fish oil, krill oil, resveratrol, and curcumin.

11. Support your immune system

At the very least, ensure that you eat healthy, get sufficient sleep, manage stress thresholds, practice proper hygiene by frequently washing your hands, and get the right nutrition to help optimum immunity.

12. Reduce inflammation

Toxicity contributes to inflammation, which leads to a heavier toxic load, which in turn prevents fat loss in return. An anti-inflammatory diet contains wild seafood, omega-3-rich plant foods, including flaxseed and chia seeds, plenty of non-starchy vegetables, and spices, including turmeric. Check with the chiropractor or other health care providers to add anti-inflammatory foods into your diet, including fish oil, krill oil, resveratrol, and curcumin.

26

13. Visit a chiropractor

Chiropractic changes influence the nervous system, which regulates all metabolic pathways and processes of detoxification. Being adapted will allow the body to detoxify and function optimally at its highest level.

Toxic overload is an often underestimated factor in obesity, and the correct detoxification strategy will supply you with the nutrition the body needs to regenerate and shed weight. Although such techniques provide a highly useful starting point, a chiropractor or other health-care practitioner may help you develop an appropriately personalized detoxification program focused on particular requirements.

14. Supplement your natural detoxification program twice a year

Although your cells are actively detoxifying, try performing a more organized detox as a full-body spring cleanse (or fall). These schedules, which usually last from two to three weeks, contain all the vitals to help optimally detoxify the liver and other organs, including protein, nutrients, and a detox-minded eating plan.

15. Other Helpful Detox Tips

Although no current research or evidence favors the use of detox diets to remove toxins from your body, some dietary changes and lifestyle habits can help lower the toxin load and improve the detoxification mechanism in your body.

Eat sulfur-containing foods. Foods that are rich in sulfur, such as onions, broccoli, and garlic, increase the excretion of heavy metals such as cadmium.

Support glutathione. Consuming sulfur-rich foods such as eggs, broccoli, and garlic helps improve the activity of glutathione, a significant antioxidant the body creates, which is heavily involved in detoxification.

Flavor dishes with cilantro. Cilantro enhances the excretion of many pollutants, including heavy metals such as lead, and contaminants like phthalates and insecticides.

Try out chlorella. According to animal research, chlorella is a form of algae that has several nutritional benefits and can enhance the elimination of pollutants, such as heavy metals.

Choose natural body care. You will also reduce the exposure to toxins by utilizing natural deodorants, make-ups, moisturizers, shampoos, and other personal care items.

While promising, several of those results were seen only in animal experiments. Hence, human studies are needed to confirm these findings. Some lifestyle and dietary improvements may enhance the natural detoxification mechanism in your body.

Switch to natural cleaning products. You will reduce the exposure to possibly harmful substances by preferring natural cleaning materials such as vinegar and baking soda over synthetic cleaning agents.

2.6 Natural Ways for Detoxification

Detox Your Body Naturally

Celebrities are particularly well recognized for extreme-leaning body detoxes (colonic irrigation, leech treatment or fasting). Not all strategy that seeks to counter the aggregation of impure substances is too serious.

Down are a number of backed and expert approaches that could help you shed toxins. You should realize that certain detox strategies have not been well tested, so it's better to let your doctor try some detoxification procedures before you start. Any individuals might be cautioned against such detox systems, for example, nursing or pregnant women and with the chronic disease.

Dry Brushing

Adopted from Ayurveda's ancient healing method, exfoliating the body and face with a natural shower gloves before getting into the shower helps in two ways: it sloughs off dead skin cells and open pores, acting as a toxin escape path. Second, the massaging activity serves to dislodge contaminants from the bloodstream of the body, priming them to eliminate. After the shower, moisturize your body with natural body oil (lathering a liquid loaded with chemicals will negate the whole purpose).

Advantages:

The methodology is swift and quick.

It assists in external and internal detoxification.

If you've invested in brushes, you do not need to buy anything else.

Eliminating Problem Foods

If you encounter signs of toxic overload, the regimen for removal (sometimes referred to as the "hypoallergenic diet") specifies that the regimen should lose the most common food sensitivities for almost a month. You can be advised by a doctor or nutritionist on what to eliminate, but often you eliminate gluten, dairy, soy, corn, poultry, sugar, and alcohol when consuming a healthier diet of whole food. The off-limited items are then introduced in one at a time to your diet to help you determine what can cause the symptoms.

Advantages:

This offers direct input into what causes adverse bodily responses.

You offer a break to sugar and processed products that are linked with the disease.

Practicing Yoga

The intense, rhythmic inhalations and yoga exhalations will take care of the parasympathetic nervous system in your body — and that enhances circulation and helps eliminate contaminants in our body's metabolism. The twisting poses, in particular, like triangle posture, are all-stars in detoxification. Sometimes compared to wringing out a dirty sponge, twisting positions strain out congestion in the lymph (the transparent lymphatic system fluid that fills the lymph nodes with internal sludge for filtration) to maintain it circulating.

Dr. Sebi Diet

Advantages:

It is healthy for your mind body and mind.

Sweat from motion will cause more detoxification.

Sweating

Evidence is inconsistent for how often pollutants escape by abruptness, but ample work has been done to thumbs up daily intense activity and brief spurts in the sauna or steam room (if they are associated with any health problems you might have). Sweat contains other poisonous elements. Some contaminants in a category called polybrominated diphenyl ethers (PBDEs) tend to be purged with perspiration. PBDEs are used as flame retardants in goods and have generally become recognized as harmful to our well-being. Just make sure with all the sweating, you remain hydrated.

Advantages:

It can be tailored to fit your timetable, location, and strength.

You are also reaping cardio's health-boosting effects.

2.7 Other Health Benefits

Your strongest reset button may be to detox the body in a safe way. It will fix the acute effects and theoretically reverse the risk of being sick down the line. Here are some positive improvements which you can find after detoxification:

Increased Energy

If you clear out toxins and waste from the body and consume detoxifying substances, expect to feel better and more energized. (Lower inflammation, improved digestion, and adequate hydration may all lead to the revitalizing effect.)

Feeling Less Stressed

You can remove certain stress factors after a body detox, including sleep debt and a diet rich in processed carbs and caffeine. Around the same time, self-care practice will

Dr. Sebi Diet

relieve the mental stress in itself. Although detoxes remove physical stress and contaminants, it is all about removing mental clutter.

Weight Loss

You are also deprived of the addiction and cravings correlated with processed diets and added sugar, which may contribute to weight gain. Less stress, coupled with improved food preference and portion awareness, will also help shed pounds.

Happier Gut

Detoxes can help cleanse the liver. We may feel gas, bloating, and constipation without having an optimally working liver.

You may have learned about "detoxifying the body," but did you do it on your own?

If you've contemplated a detox but aren't positive, hearing about the various advantages of detoxification can help you make up your mind. Detox diets help getting rid of the body from contaminants and developing behaviors that can hold you on track for a healthy life. As you might know, the body has its own normal forms of detoxification. Liver, sweat, and urine are all means of ridding the body of contaminants. But these vital organs often function too intensely and need a rest. A detox diet is a perfect way to release the organs from the strain, and you can maintain them healthy for the future.

2.8 Types of Detox Diets

There are many myriad forms of detox diets, and each can show you slightly different outcomes. But no matter what you want, there's no questioning about the effects of detoxification. Let us have a peek at 10 forms; you might benefit from a detox diet.

1. Weight Loss and Management

Besides dropping weight, there are other causes to undergo a detox. But if weight reduction is one of your priorities, a detox diet may be an ideal way to begin your change. The detoxification will also assist in weight management in the long run. Use a diet to get your body on board whether you are at an optimum weight but want to

Dr. Sebi Diet

make sure that you remain there. One of the great aspects of a detox is that it's not about improving right now — it's setting you up to develop good practices to come. And just after detoxing, you still have the routines you need to maintain track of potential weight loss or weight maintenance.

2. More Energy

An energy increase is one of the first perks you'll find after detoxifying. Who doesn't want to get more energy through the day? The modern world needs a lot from us, between jobs, families, leisure, exercise, and social life. Detoxifying removes things like sugar and caffeine away that trigger energy drops, leaving you with more healthy resources all day long.

3. Aids Internal Organs

As described above, detoxing helps eliminate toxins from your body. It purifies contaminants that might not be able to keep up with the bodies and provides a much-needed break to those organs that are responsible for eliminating waste.

Even if the liver, kidneys, and other organs function well, the body can often contain more contaminants than you know. A detox is a perfect way to get rid of certain contaminants to more efficiently support the internal organs do their work.

4. Better Immune System

Because detoxification reduces some of the stress from your organs, they can then do a better job of defending your body from disease. You'll consume much-needed nutrients more easily, including vitamin C, proven to be helpful for the immune system.

If you are on a detox that involves taking some herbs, you may experience a boost to the lymphatic system as well. This program is partially responsible for keeping you healthy and free from contaminants, so you'll want it to perform well.

5. Nicer Breath

Your body's elimination of contaminants has several pleasant side effects, besides enhancing your well-being. Good breath is among the advantages of detoxification. It will allow the digestive system to work properly, eliminating some of the triggers of bad breath.

Bear in mind, though, that during detox, your breath can potentially get worse because your body responds to the changes and removes toxins. You can see the results when it's complete.

6. Clearer Skin

You may have even the most advanced skincare routines, but you can always encounter skin issues if your food isn't clean. One of the surefire methods to clean the skin is by detox. Some detoxes also have a sauna feature, so that you can actually sweat out some of the contaminants that clutter your pores. But even though you are using just food, you can always get effects.

As with your intake, the issue often gets worse during the detox itself, then clear up after the detox has completed. So brace yourself for a sudden breakout or skin problem when your body is in the process of detox.

7. Improved Thinking

Detoxing is the way to go, with clearer thinking and a stronger memory. The benefits of detoxification are not mere physical benefits. Many detoxes also provide strategies to take control of your mind, as well as the body. For starters, you might be using meditation as part of your detox program.

You could also be impacted by sugar crashes and other adverse consequences of an unhealthy diet. If the detox benefit has been felt, you may never want to go back.

8. Shinier Hair

Shiny, smooth hair is another benefit of detoxification. For the development of healthier hair, the follicles need the right nutrients. Toxin accumulation stops certain nutrients from reaching where they need to go and also contributes to brittle, delicate, torn tresses.

Dr. Sebi Diet

You could see quicker development, too, making this a perfect opportunity for someone looking to grow their hair.

9. Slowed Signs of Aging

It's a good thing to get older, but we don't necessarily like the visible symptoms of aging that come with it.

By reducing the usage of toxins that contribute to the skin damage we usually associate with growing older, detoxing helps you slow down visible signs of aging.

10. Enjoy Your Food

Most of the misconceptions about detoxification are that during the procedure, you do not like something that you ingest. The truth is a healthy diet will also make you appreciate your diet more. That does not suggest you're not going to feel sugar cravings and the other items you're leaving out of your diet — at least at first.

But detoxification enhances your link with, and awareness of, the stuff that you place in your body. You should be deliberately preparing balanced, well-rounded meals, so you will also use some of the items that you enjoy whilst adding different products that you may come to love as well.

2.9 Dangerous Detox Side Effects

At most, detox items and diets do not impact the well-being of individuals to a significant degree, and that gives them any limited positive benefits. At worst, the detox goods will damage the body somewhat.

One of the problems of detox craze is that approaches are mostly unregulated and untested. You could purchase anything quickly and might end up being toxic to the body.

If you are considering taking a detox diet, you could change your mind after discovering the harmful ways that your body could be impacted.

Dehydration

It's not unusual to use laxatives or diuretics for certain detox programs, and people use more of the restroom.

When doctors offer those drugs and taking them over a limited period of time, they are healthy. But it may contribute to extreme dehydration as people take them for long stretches of time.

Dehydration is more about simply getting to use additional fluids. Over time, dehydration can trigger significant harm to major organs or can contribute to more severe health problems such as seizures.

Stomach Problems

Detox pills and diets can use a variety of substances to "purge" toxins in the body. The laxatives, supplements, and even the "helpful" bacteria contained in some of such items may cause severe gastrointestinal problems.

Many individuals with diarrhea, nausea, and vomiting may experience issues with detox diets and cleanse.

Nutrient Deficiencies

A number of detox diets include people removing those products that are believed to induce toxin build-up.

Many people eliminate meat and dairy without any complications from their foods, but that is generally combined with modifying their recipes to make up for the loss of nutrients.

Many of these detox diets entail taking out of your diet essential nutrients without providing a healthy means of replacing them. If you practice detox diets, you may lose out on essential vitamins and minerals.

Highly Restrictive

Detox diets usually are considered to be highly stringent, but the degree to which foods and drinks are limited differs. Some plans require you to eat just a few hundred calories, while some plans require you to ingest enough food to meet the entire day's energy requirements. The lowest calorie detox diets are those that simply provide liquid or juice diets.

There are detox plans, for example, that limit the consumption many times a day to only a lemon or tea drink. This detox system, also named the "master cleanse," recommends you consume a quarter of saltwater in the morning and a cup of any herbal laxative tea in the evening before bed. You drink a very low calorie "lemonade" consisting of lemons, maple syrup, cayenne pepper, and a few other ingredients during daytime hours.

If you adopt the master cleanse plan, you are only able to eat between 500 and 700 calories a day, much smaller than most adults will consider. Extremely low-calorie diets like this are usually advised only under professional supervision as there is a chance of risks in the well-being, particularly if you are overweight or obese.

Another downside to following an extremely restricted diet is the possibility it could backfire. Indeed, multiple reports, including one reported in the Neuroscience Journal, referring to the extreme caloric restriction as a dietary trend that encourages binge eating.

Safety Concerns

Aside from issues created by inadequate food consumption, there are other health risks that people may be mindful of while following a detox diet. Potential safety threats exist, according to the National Center for Complementary and Integrative Health.

For starters, whether they drink too much juice or don't get enough nutrients, persons with other medical problems, including diabetes or kidney failure, might be affected. Additionally, persons with a history of a stomach illness, bowel cancer, renal failure, or cardiac disorder do not take detox diets that require treatments for colon cleansing.

Dr. Sebi Diet

Juice diets cannot be healthy and allow you to purchase specific items. Juices that have not been preserved or otherwise handled to eliminate harmful bacteria may make people sick, including children, the elderly, and those with weakened immune systems.

Finally, not all detox selling services have truthful facts regarding their goods. The FDA and the FTC took action against many businesses marketing detox/cleansing drugs because they included additives that were prohibited or actually dangerous, and they were sold with misleading statements or were advertised for improper use.

Programs Lack Scientific Support

There is a shortage of high-quality, unbiased research that endorse the usage of detox diets. Studies that endorse such diets are mostly supported by a company that offers a treatment plan that is restricted in nature or operates on rodents.

There are also some reports that challenge the need for a detox diet.

For example, in one published report,9 authors of the analysis challenged the need for some specific diet to remove synthetic chemicals (called POPs or persistent organic pollutants) that accumulate in human adipose tissue.

"There is still no medical opinion as to why existing rates of sensitivity to POPs are harmful to human safety, which leaves it uncertain if removing them will provide any benefits. The detox industry works under the premise that the amount of a foreign chemical in the body would be a source of alarm, but this idea is unsubstantiated. "Even though such diets were sufficient to decrease the amounts of harmful contaminants in the body, the effects will be impossible to be observable.

The research reported in The Journal of Alternative and Complementary Medicine 10 explored the usage in the United States of therapeutic detoxification treatments operated by registered naturopathic doctors (NDs). Study authors observed that while most NDs utilized such follow-up measures during detoxification therapy, none offered quantitative evaluation to assess the efficacy of treatment.

And research participants who see a small gain also say findings are short-lived.

Dr. Sebi Diet

One research reported in Current Gastroenterology Reports contrasted various diets, showing that "Juicing or detoxification diets appear to function as they yield incredibly low caloric consumption for brief periods of time, but continue to contribute to weight gain until a regular diet is restored."

Reduced Energy

Extreme exhaustion is a common concern that many people who go on detox diets have shared. Poor calorie consumption is possibly a primary source. Many detox diets that restrict or totally exclude the consumption of carbohydrates are often likely to induce exhaustion because carbohydrates provide rapid energy for the body.

Such very-low-calorie plans may often cause headaches, fainting, fatigue, dehydration, and hunger pangs, and detox programs that contain laxatives may trigger extreme enough diarrhea to result in dehydration and electrolyte imbalances.

Expensive

Not all detox diets are costly, but there are others that allow you to purchase packs or entire sets like supplements. The final price may be substantial.

For example, one package that lasts 10 days requires three bottles of supplement tablets, one bottle of cherry juice, and a shake mix. The rate is $249, with no shipping. A famous three-day raw juice cleanse will set you back $99, and it can cost approximately $400 for a longer 90-day program that offers cell detoxification.

When you realize the minimal advantages such services are likely to offer, many customers will get the idea that it is not worth the expense.

The Bottom Line

Most nutrition experts and wellness organizations are not advocating detox diets. Such short-lived, yet very minimal meal schemes have several pitfalls. The body is also doing a fine job at cleaning away contaminants. The type of detox effects that you may receive through foods and items are serious enough to make someone think twice before doing so. Urge anyone who is interested in weight loss and their body being "purified" to eat well and exercise. That's more than enough to improve your body and your health.

Chapter 3: Disease Reversal with Detoxification and Cleansing

This chapter discusses that how detoxification and cleansing procedures help in preventing serious health problems. As liver and digestive system are the main organs that deal with the toxins present in the body so to make them work efficiently detoxification and cleansing approaches are mandatory. This chapters gives the insight about how liver and digestive issues lead to the toxins build up in the body, what are their symptoms and how they can be minimized to attain good health. Liver and digestive system are the main organs for the breakdown and removal of toxic compounds from the body.

3.1 How does detox help prevent potential diseases?

Human anatomy has been designed to lead a balanced life in an exceptional way, but owing to our chaotic, sometimes out of control "modern world lifestyle," and its environment, our bodies, and minds are subject to a constant influx of toxins. Our body functions are at considerable risk under this strain because they are sometimes weakened and may quickly cede to diseases and illnesses. A detox is like pressing a reset button on the body. This gives a break to our bodies and brains and slows down the digestive tract. Our bodies go into recovery mode after detox, so we can concentrate on self-care and healing.

What does your liver do?

The liver is the largest organ of the body at about 1.4 kg and conducts a variety of important functions, including:

• Helps produce vitamin D required to produce hormones

• Removes toxic chemicals, microbes and unwanted hormones from the body

• Stores vitamins and minerals that include iron and vitamin B12 as well

• Processes the fats, proteins, and carbohydrates from the food you consume so you can get the energy and nutrients from whatever you consume

Dr. Sebi Diet

• Creates products that are used by your immune system to protect your body from infections.

• Stores the sugar (glycogen) for future use when energy is required by your body

Thus you can see, your liver, and your hormonal well-being, is incredibly essential to your overall health. If it doesn't perform well, you need to take the measures to help detoxify your liver and regain its healthy function. What you consume, drink, but even breathe and come in touch with through your skin, and it then reaches your bloodstream, the body needs to process it. So maintaining a balanced lifestyle and adopting a healthy diet is incredibly essential to your well-being, especially your liver's health and well-being.

Symptoms of toxic liver

Now the liver is metabolizing the hormones and other compounds through what is known as phase 1 and phase 2 pathways, two main stages.

If your blood is very toxic, it can have a detrimental impact on your liver's well-being, and you might be suffering from what's considered a congested liver.

Symptoms with badly clogged liver include:

- Hormonal imbalance
- Weight gain
- Skin issues of rosacea, acne, dermatitis, rashes, psoriasis, and eczema
- Exhaustion
- Impaired digestion
- Chemical sensitivities

And possibly inflammation in the upper right portion of the abdomen where the liver is situated.

Fatty liver disease

Dr. Sebi Diet

Furthermore, you will increase your risk of dying from what is considered non-alcoholic fatty liver disease from an unhealthy diet and lifestyle, which is when you get so much fat in your liver. The fatty liver disorder is now America's most prevalent form of dreadful liver disease, affecting 70 million Americans — that's one in three people.

It may contribute to hepatic cancer, liver disease, and death at its worst. The warning factors for fatty liver disease now include:

- Type 2 diabetes and pre-diabetes
- Being overweight
- Possessing elevated amounts of fat in the body, such as cholesterol and triglycerides
- Recovering from other diseases, such as hepatitis C
- Exposure to contaminants
- Metabolic syndrome
- High blood pressure

Research has been conducted on 9,000 American people who have been followed for about 13 years. It showed that there is a close correlation between consumption of cholesterol (from the diet they consume, including, for example, animal products such as eggs and meat) and hospitalization and mortality from liver cancer and cirrhosis. That is how dietary cholesterol can oxidize, creating harmful and carcinogenic consequences. So consuming animal products is another way the liver will sustain damage, and that may lead to liver cirrhosis (liver scarring) and even hepatic cancer.

3.2 How to detox for digestive issues

The Role Played by Toxins in Your Digestion Issues

Our lives are jammed full of ever more dangerous chemicals. Our food, domestic cleaners, cosmetics, self-care products, and the air itself have environmental pollutants. Today only low-grade contaminants occur on most typically cultivated vegetables and fruits.

Dr. Sebi Diet

Healthy bodies detoxify all that may be dangerous to eliminate. Yet over time, we're subjected to the contaminants and pollutants that are formed in our bodies and inflict harmful effects. The contaminants in your body will trigger your digestive system to quit functioning properly, resulting in gaining weight and a host of other problems.

What happens if the digestive system doesn't operate properly?

If your digestive tract is not operating well, contaminants overload the liver. Some contaminants can live long, which can make us feel ill and lethargic. The metabolism of the body slows down, and the accumulation of contaminants triggers fluid accumulation, bloating and puffiness before you realize it.

Symptoms:

- Gas / Burping
- Sore skin
- Leaky intestine
- Heartburn
- Weight increase
- Bloating
- Stomach discomfort
- Persistent swelling
- Constipation
- Nausea
- Appetite loss
- Diarrhea and vomiting
- Extreme fatigue
- Mental distress
- Low-grade diseases
- Puffy or bags around the eyes
- Allergies

How Toxins Lead To Digestive Problems

The more contaminants you encounter in your life, the more detrimental effects body parts face. Your Food and environment decide how high your toxic load is over time, and then the toxicity triggers inflammation, which contributes to gain weight.

How these toxins induce digestive problems is a complex procedure, which mainly happens in your liver which is responsible for transforming contaminants into extremely reactive metabolites before these contaminants are fully excreted from the body. Although your body's liver is most damaged by toxins –gallbladder, intestines and pancreas are all important organs that retain toxins in your digestive system.

A healthy digestive processes break down the diet to absorb the necessary vitamins and minerals that they can to expel the unusable products in your everyday bowel movements. If this one-way mechanism will not function well, people more commonly experience:

- Nausea
- Leaky gut
- Indigestion
- Diarrhea
- Irritable bowel syndrome
- Constipation

If the symptoms linger, an unstable digestive tract is often correlated with:

- Allergies, mainly in food
- Hemorrhoids
- Obesity and weight gain
- Dehydration
- Nutrient deficiencies
- Diabetes
- Ulcers
- Small intestinal overgrowth

Dr. Sebi Diet

- Persistent diarrhea

- Signs of liver disease

- Skin issues like Psoriasis or Eczema

- Hemolytic uremic syndrome

- Brain and Heart problems

- Autoimmune conditions, like Multiple Sclerosis, Crohn's Disease, Celiac Disease, Lupus, Rheumatoid Arthritis and more

How to Treat Issues related to Digestive tract Caused by Toxins

The best way to cure digestive issues induced by contaminants is to eliminate or reduce the intake, to clear toxic accumulation from the body.

There are also different methods that you should seek to rid the body of contaminants before they induce stomach problems. Full body detoxification is also effective remedies for toxin-induced digestive disorders, whereas other alternative approaches such as consuming the correct foods and utilizing supplements to enhance gastrointestinal well-being can help.

Your body, though, can only detoxify adequately with the correct food, lots of sleep, and good hygiene.

Paybacks of Detox for Digestive Issues

A digestive detox uses natural foods to wash away contaminants from the body. Digestive health is important to your well-being, so you can find advantages by cleansing up your body:

- Intestines

- Colon

- Liver

Detoxes can remove the body's toxic substances so pollutants until the pounds pile up. They improve your digestive well-being, too. Any contaminants within you will normally grow removed before they have enough time to inflict damage.

Dr. Sebi Diet

A detox cleanse can help with loss of weight and support certain causes contributing to obesity, such as persistent inflammation. Specialists often consider that certain chronic diseases of proper digestive hygiene are easy to prevent.

People also feel more active following detox and have restored vigor. Since stress and contaminants impair the regular operation of the body, you might start feeling like your old self and bouncing back into good health.

Some Other Advantages of Detoxing For Digestion

Detox can also help in cleaning the large intestine or liver, where the healthy bacteria breakdown the food. Also, colon cleansing assists in other stomach disorders, such as constipation and abnormal bowel movements. So, it can also reduce the chances of colon cancer. By eating foods such as leafy greens and broccoli may help detoxify the colon, of course.

Digestive Problems and Detox Strategies

Be aware of what's going through your body when it comes to seeking treatment for stomach disorders that are perfect for your needs. For your digestive well-being, your dietary patterns, food nutrients, and detox remedies all play a role. For you, the right approach will also rely on your living style.

Many people consume more vegetables or nuts than products that are refined. Some use other foods to cleanse their bodies as laxatives. Natural remedies such as ginger or apple cider vinegar can help with negative symptoms. In fact, people use detox foods to remove contaminants from the body, varying from juice fasts to supplements or diuretics. Cleanses are also eligible for sale to disinfect either the entire body or a particular area, such as the colon.

Chapter 4: Dr. Sebi Approved Herbs and Food Items

This chapter highlights the main rules to follow the diet designed by Dr. Sebi. These are the strict rules that must be followed and that are to eliminate all the dairy and meat products from diet, only allowed foods can be consumed, seedless fruits or vegetables cannot be eaten by a person following this diet. Also this chapter includes the detailed list of all the herbs along with the parts of the herb that is allowed to be consumed. Each food group with the permitted items are also mentioned. These are the food items that help to alkalize the body because it is believed that acidic body will lead to the occurrence of other diseases.

4.1 Dr. Sebi Diet Rules

You must observe these main guidelines, according to Dr. Sebi's dietary guide:

Rule 1. You just have to consume foods specified in the nutritional manual.

Rule 2. Drink 1 gallon (3.8 liters) of water daily.

Rule 3. Take the supplements by Dr. Sebi one hour before taking medications.

Rule 4. No animal products are allowed.

Rule 5. Alcohol is not allowed.

Rule 6. Avoid wheat goods, and use only the "natural grains" specified in the guide.

Rule 7. Avoid using a microwave to keep the food from being poisoned.

Rule 8. Eliminate fruits that are canned or seedless.

There are no clear rules on the nutrients. This diet is poor in protein, though, as it excludes beans, lentils, and meat and soy foods. Protein is an essential effective nutrient for strong muscles, skin, and joints.

In fact, you're supposed to purchase cell food items from Dr. Sebi, which are supplements that aim to clean the body and nourish the cells.

It is advised to buy the "all-inclusive" bundle, which contains 20 separate items promising to cleanse up and rebuild the whole body at the quickest possible pace.

Besides this, there are no clear guidelines for the supplements. Instead, you can order some medication that fits your health issues.

The "Bio Ferro" pills, for example, promise to cure liver issues, cleanse the blood, improve immunity, encourage weight loss, aid digestion disorders, and enhance general well-being.

Additionally, the products do not include a full list of nutrients or their proportions, rendering it impossible to determine whether they can fulfill the everyday requirements.

Summary

Dr. Sebi's diet has eight main rules to fulfill. They concentrate mainly on eliminating animal products, ultra-processed food, and taking the patented supplements.

4.2 What does it mean to alkalize the body?

An alkaline diet is focused on the idea that the food you consume regulates the body's pH. Because the products that our body utilizes leave behind metabolic waste, the theory is that the waste will have a pH that ranges from alkaline to acidic.

In various areas, the human body has varying pH ratios, with organs such as the stomach becoming more acidic, whereas blood becomes more alkaline. One of the body products that is specifically influenced by the foods we consume is pee, which is a sensor in the blood to regulate pH.

The larger group of "alkaline diets" is focused around the topic of metabolic waste, and one of those is the Dr. Sebi diet. They are strong enough to promote consuming healthy plant-based foods. However, there is no study behind alkalizing the body, and the arguments made are not backed by evidence.

Dr. Sebi Diet

4.3 Dr. Sebi Approved Herbs List

Anamu/Guinea Hen Weed: Whole Herb

Arnica: Root, Flower

Basil: Leaf, Essential Oil

Bay leaves: Leaf

Bladderwrack: Whole Herb

Blue Vervain: Leaf, Flower

Bugleweed: Aerial parts

Burdock: Root

Catnip: Aerial Parts

Cancansa/Cansasa/Red Willow Bark: Bark

Cannabis (Marijuana/Hemp): Flower, leaf, seed, stem

Capadula: Bark, Root

Cardo Santo/Blessed Thistle/Holy Thistle: Aerial Part

Cascara Sagrada/Sacred Bark: Bark

Cayenne/African Bird Pepper: Fruit

Centaury/Star Thistle/Knapweed: Flowering Aerial Parts

Chamomile: Flower, Leaf

Chaparro Amargo: Leaf, Branch

Chickweed: Whole Herb

Clove: Undeveloped Flower Bud

Cocolmeca: Root

Condurango: Vine, Bark

Contribo/Birthwort: Root, Aerial Part

Dr. Sebi Diet

Cordoncillo Negro: Bark

Cuachalalate: Bark

Dandelion: Root, Leaf (Mainly root used as medicine)

Drago/Dracaeana Draco/Dragon Tree: Leaf, Bark

Elderberry: Berry, Flower

Eucalyptus: Leaf

Eyebright: Aerial Parts

Fennel: Seed

Feverfew/Santa Maria: Whole Plant, Root, Flowering & Fruiting

Flor de Manita/Hand Flower Tree: Flower

Ginger: Root

Guaco/Mikania: Root

Governadora/Chaparral: Leaf/Flower

Hoodia Gordonii/Kalahari Cactus: Fleshy part of the stem

Hombre Grande/Quassia/Bitter Wood: Bark

Hortensia/Hydrangea: Dried Rhizome, Root

Huereque/Wereke: Root

Iboga: Root Bark

Kalawalla: Rhizome, Frond, Leaf

Kinkeliba/Seh Haw: Leaf, Root, and Bark

Lavender: Flower, Leaves

Lemon Verbena: Leaves, Flowering Top

Lily of the Valley: Flower

Linden: Flower

Dr. Sebi Diet

Lirio/Lily: Flower, Bulb, Leaf

Locust: Bark

Lupulo/Hops: Flower

Manzo: Root, Rhizome, Leaf

Marula: Bark, Fruit, Leaf, Kernel, Nut

Milk Thistle: Seed

Mullein/Gordolobo: Flower, leaf, seed, stem

Myrrh: Resin

Nopal: Cactus

Oak Bark / Encino: Bark

Ortiga/Stinging Nettle: Leaf

Pavana/Croton: Seed

Pao Periera: Bark, Stem

Palo Mulato: Bark

Peony: Root, Root Bark

Pinguicula/Butterwort: Leaf

Prodigiosa/Bricklebush/Leaf of Life: Leaf

Prunella Vulgaris / Self-Heal: Whole Herb

Purslane/Verdolaga: Leaf, Young Shoot, Stem

Red Clover: Flower

Red Raspberry: Leaf

Rhubarb: Root

Salsify/Goatsbeard/Oyster Plant: Root, Leaves, Flower, Seed, Young Stem

San Pedro Cactus: Whole Herb

Dr. Sebi Diet

Santa Maria/Sage: Leaf

Sapo/Saponaire/Hierba del Sapo/Mexican Thistle: Whole Herb

Sarsaparilla: Root

Sea Moss: Seaweed

Sempervivum/Houseleek: Leaf, Leaf Sap

Sensitiva/Shameplant/Dead and Wake: Dried Whole Plant, Root, Leaf, Seed

Senecio/Groundsel/Ragwort: Whole Herb

Soursop: Leaf

Shepherd's Purse: Whole Herb

Shiny Bush Plant/Pepper Elder: Root, Aerial Part

Tila/Linden: Flower

Tronadora: Leaf, Stem

Turnera/Damiana: Leaf

Valeriana/Valerian: Root

Yarrow/Queen Anne's lace: Aerial Part, Essential Oil

Yellowdock: Root

Yohimbe: Whole Herb

4.4 Dr. Sebi Approved Food Items from each Food Groups

Dr. Sebi Vegetable List

As for all his electric products, Dr. Sebi claimed that people could consume products other than GMOs. That involves fruits and vegetables rendered seedless or modified to produce more minerals and vitamins than naturally, they do. Dr. Sebi's vegetable list is very broad and varied, with lots of choices for making multiple diverse meals. This list contains:

Dr. Sebi Diet

- Arame
- Amaranth
- Bell Pepper
- Avocado
- Cherry and Plum Tomato
- Chayote
- Cucumber
- Dulse
- Dandelion Greens
- Hijiki
- Garbanzo Beans
- Kale
- Izote flower and leaf
- Mushrooms except for Shitake
- Lettuce except for iceberg
- Nori
- Okra
- Nopales
- Olives
- Purslane Verdolaga
- Tomatillo
- Onions
- Sea Vegetables
- Squash
- Turnip Greens
- Wakame
- Watercress
- Zucchini
- Wild Arugula

Dr. Sebi Diet

Dr. Sebi Fruit List

While the list of vegetables is lengthy, the list of fruits is vey restrict, and certain varieties of fruits are not allow for the consumption when on a diet by Dr. Sebi. However, the selection of fruits is still providing a broad range of choices to diet followers. For example, on Dr. Sebi's food list, all kinds of berries are permitted besides cranberries, which is a fruit made by man. The list also includes:

- Bananas
- Berries
- Apples
- Currants
- Dates
- Figs
- Cantaloupe
- Cherries
- Grapes
- Limes
- Mango
- Prunes
- Raisins
- Soft Jelly Coconuts
- Melons
- Peaches
- Pears
- Plums
- Prickly Pear
- Sour soups
- Orange
- Papayas

- Tamarind

Dr. Sebi Food List Spices and Seasonings

- Bay Leaf
- Cayenne
- Cloves
- Achiote
- Basil
- Dill
- Oregano
- Habanero
- Powdered Granulated Seaweed
- Onion Powder
- Tarragon
- Thyme
- Pure Sea Salt
- Sweet Basil
- Sage
- Savory

Alkaline Grains

- Kamut
- Amaranth
- Fonio
- Quinoa
- Tef
- Rye
- Spelt
- Wild Rice

Alkaline Sugars and Sweeteners

- Coconut Sugar
- 100% Pure Agave Syrup from cactus
- Date Sugar from dried dates

Dr. Sebi Herbal Teas

- Elderberry
- Ginger
- Red Raspberry
- Burdock
- Chamomile
- Fennel
- Tila

Nuts and Seeds

- Walnuts
- Brazil Nuts
- Hemp seeds
- Raw Sesame Seeds

Oils

- Olive Oil
- Coconut Oil
- Grapeseed Oil
- Sesame Oil
- Hempseed Oil
- Avocado Oil

Dr. Sebi Diet

Chapter 5: Recipes

This chapter consists of the lots of recipes that can be cooked with such a low number of allowed food items. As these are the vegan food items and the dishes made of these food items are perfect for a vegetarian. There are the recipes for main dishes, salads, milk alternatives, soups, desserts, sauces, dips, butter, cheese, smoothies, shakes and juices. These are the recipes enough to follow for a longer period of time.

5.1 Main Dishes

Chickpea Burger

This recipe will make 3-4 burgers.

Ingredients

- 1 cup Garbanzo Bean Flour
- 1/2 cup Diced Onions
- 1/2 cup Green Peppers, Diced
- 1/2 cup Kale, Diced
- 1 Plum Tomato, Diced
- 2 Tsp. Basil
- 2 tsp. Oregano
- 2 tsp. Powdered onion
- 2 tsp. Sea Salt
- 1 tsp. Dill
- 1/2 tsp. Powdered ginger
- Grape seed oil
- 1/2 tsp. Cayenne Pepper
- 1/4-1/2 cup Spring Water

Directions

1. Mix all seasonings and vegetables together in a big bowl, then combine them in the flour.

2. Little by little add water and blend before the mixture can turn into a patty. Should it be too soft, put more flour.

3. Add oil to skillet, and cook on medium-high heat the patties on either side for 2-3 minutes. Continue to turn until both sides are brown.

4. Serve and devour your Alkaline Chickpea Burgers on alkaline flatbread!

Alkaline Pizza Crust

Ingredients

- 1 1/2 cup Spelt Flour
- 1 tsp. Powdered onion
- 1 tsp. Oregano
- 2 tsp. Sesame
- 1 tsp. Sea Salt
- 2 tsp. Agave
- 2 tsp. Grapeseed Oil
- 1 cup Spring water

Directions

1. Preheat oven to 400 ° F.

2. In a medium sized container, combine all of the ingredients together, including only 1/2 cup of spring water. Slowly pour water before the dough can be formed into a ball; if too much water is used pour more flour.

3. Coat the baking sheet thinly with grape seed oil, apply flour to your hands and roll the dough out onto the baking sheet.

4. Brush with grape seed oil to the tip of the crust and stab holes with a fork into it. Bake crust for 10-15 minutes.

5. Prepare the pizza sauce with tomato or avocado as the crust bakes. 6. Add the pizza sauce, brazil nut cheese *, mushrooms, chili peppers, and onions after the crust is cooked. 15-20 minutes to bake the pizza.

6. Enjoy your Alkaline Veggie Pizza!

* Nut cheese helps to cook the toppings during the baking process. If you don't have some nut cheese, prefer to sauté the toppings before baking.

Vegan Alkaline Ribs

This recipe will make 1 serving per mushroom.

Ingredients

- 2 portobello mushrooms
- 1/2 cup alkaline barbecue sauce
- 1/4 cup spring water
- 1 tsp. Sea salt
- 1 tsp. Powdered onion
- 1/2 tsp. cayenne
- Grapeseed oil
- Basting brush
- Cast-iron griddle
- Skewers (optional)

This dish may also be served on a grill, cooked in a skillet or cooked at 350 degrees F for 10-15 minutes (after step 4).

You can also cook the mushrooms like riblets, if you don't have skewers.

Directions

1. Scrape gills off each mushroom cap's underside to prevent an earthy flavor, then slice mushrooms about 1/2 inch apart.

Dr. Sebi Diet

2. Add mushrooms to a wide pot then add seasonings, water, then barbecue sauce for the most part.

3. Cover with a lid, shake and keep for around 6-8 hours in the refrigerator. Flip the container after 2 hours.

4. Take a skewer and pass around the center by 3 mushrooms, add the other skewer, then attach another 2-3 more pieces. You should cook these as riblets if some slices fall.

5. Spray the griddle with oil over medium heat and cook the ribs for 12-15 minutes, tossing after 3 minutes. Brush with more barbecue sauce, if a few more flips are desired.

Alkaline Electric Sloppy Joe

This recipe makes 4-6 servings.

Ingredients

- 2 cups of cooked spelt or kamut
- 1 cup of cooked garbanzo beans
- 1 1/2 cup of Alkaline Barbecue sauce
- 1/2 cup of onion
- 1/2 cup of green peppers
- 1 cup of plum tomato,
- 1 tsp. Powder of onion
- 1 tsp. of sea salt
- 1/8 tsp. Cayenne powder
- Grapeseed oil
- Food processor

Directions

1. In food processor, put the spelt and garbanzo beans and process for around 10-15 seconds.

Dr. Sebi Diet

2. Add oil and sauté onions, peppers, and seasonings in a large skillet over medium-high heat for 3-5 minutes.

3. Mix sauce with pulsed ingredients, tomato, and barbecue and cook for about 5 minutes.

4. Serve on Alkaline Flatbread and enjoy!

Alkaline Electric Flatbread

This recipe makes 4 - 6 servings.

Ingredients

- 2 cups Flour spelt
- 2 tbsp. Grapeseed oil
- 3/4 cup Spring Water
- 1 tbsp. Sea salt
- 2 tsp. Oregano
- 2 tsp. Basil
- 2 tsp. Powdered onion
- 1/4 tsp. Cayenne

Plus point of this recipe is that in only 20 minutes you can do this and it's perfect for sandwiches, wraps or mini pizzas!

Directions

1. Mix flour and seasonings together, until well blended.

2. In the mixture, add in oil and around 1/2 cup of water. Mix in water gradually, until it turns into a ball.

3. Add the flour to the workspace and knead the dough for around 5 minutes, then split it into 6 equal portions.

4. Roll out each ball into circles measuring about 4 inches.

5. Put it on medium-high heat in an ungreased skillet, tossing until ready every 2-3 minutes.

6. Enjoy your Alkaline Flatbread!

Alkaline Electric Meatloaf

Ingredients

- 3 cups Mushrooms, sliced
- 2 cups Cooked Garbanzo Beans
- 2/3 cup Alkaline Barbecue Sauce or Alkaline Ketchup
- 1 1/2 cup Garbanzo Bean Flour
- 1 cup White Onions, chopped
- 1 cup Green Peppers, chopped
- 1 Roma tomato, chopped
- 1 tsp. Agave
- 2 tbsp. Onion powder
- 1 tbsp. Sea salt
- 1 tbsp. Basil
- 1 tsp. Oregano
- 2 tsp. Savory
- 1 tsp. powdered ginger
- 1/2 tsp. Cayenne Powder
- Food processor

Directions

1. Blend mushrooms and garbanzo beans together for 30 seconds in food processor.

2. Process for 1 minute or until fully blended in seasonings, agave, 1/2 cup of white onions, 1/2 cup of green peppers and 1/3 cup barbecue sauce.

3. In a large bowl, add the mixture and mix in 1/3 cup of onions, 1/3 cup of peppers and 1 cup of flour. If the mixture is too moist put more flour.

Dr. Sebi Diet

4. Bake in oven for 35-45 minutes at 350 F.

5. Allow at least 30 minutes to cool before cutting into meatloaf or it may be mushy and fall apart.

6. Enjoy your Electric Alkaline meatloaf

Alkaline Electric Burro Mashed "Potatoes"

This recipe makes 4-6 servings.

Ingredients

- 6-8 Green Burro Bananas * or 2 cups Cooked Garbanzo Beans
- 1 cup Hemp Milk or Walnut Milk
- 2 tsp. Powder onion
- 2 tsp. Sea Salt
- 1/4 cup Green Onions, diced with Alkaline Gravy (Optional)

* Make sure that the skin is still green while preparing this dish, because it may taste sweet when the skin turns yellow. There's even a faint hint of banana as it's made with burros.

Directions

1. Split off the ends of each burro, cut each side through the skin, extract the flesh and add to the processor.

2. Pour the milk and seasonings into the food processor and blend for 1-2 minutes, then add spring water if the mixture becomes too thick.

3. Add mixture and green onions to a pan, and cook over medium heat.

4. Cook while stirring continuously for 25-30 minutes, adding more water when it becomes too dense.

5. Serve, with Alkaline Gravy!

Alkaline Electric Mushroom & Onion Gravy

Dr. Sebi Diet

This recipe will make around 2-3 cups of gravy, depending on the amount of water used.

Ingredients

- 2 - 3 cups Spring Water
- 1/2 cup Mushrooms*
- 1/2 cup Onions
- 1/4 tsp. Cayenne
- 3 tbs. Garbanzo bean flour
- 2 tbs. Grapeseed Oil
- 1 tsp. Sea Salt
- 1/2 tsp. Thyme
- 1 tsp. Onion Powder
- 1/2 tsp. Oregano

*You can skip the mushrooms if you want.

Directions

1. Add grapeseed oil over medium to high heat to fry pan

2. Sauté mushrooms & onions for A minute

3. Add all seasonings and spices except cayenne

4. Sautee for Five minutes

5. Add 2 cups of spring water

6. Add ground cayenne

7. Mix all ingredients completely and bring to a boil

8. Continue sifting a little at a time the flour, and mix with a whisk to avoid lumps

9. Start cooking until boiling, including remaining water if needed

10. Enjoy Kamut with your Alkaline Mushroom & Onion Gravy, or your favorite meal!

Alkaline Electric Spicy Kale

This makes about 4 servings.

Ingredients

- 1 bunch of Kale
- 1/4 cup Onion, diced
- 1/4 cup Red Pepper, diced
- 1 tsp. Crushed Red Pepper
- 1/4 tsp. Sea Salt
- Alkaline "Garlic" Oil or Grape Seed Oil
- Salad Spinner (optional)*

*If you do not have a salad spinner, allow kale to air dry.

Directions

1. Rinse off the kale, then fold in half per leaf, then cut off the base.

2. Chop the kale into bite-sized bits and use salad spinner to drain water.

3. Add approx. 2 tbsp. Oil to wok over high heat.

4. Stir in onions and peppers for 2-3 minutes.

5. Reduce heat to low, add the kale to the wok and cover for 5 minutes with a lid.

6. Add crushed red pepper, mix and cover with lid for an additional 3 minutes or until tender.

7. Enjoy the Spicy Kale, Alkaline!

Nori-Burritos

Ingredients

- 1 avocado, ripe
- 450 gr. cucumber (seeded)
- 1/2 mango, ripe
- 4 sheets nori seaweed

Dr. Sebi Diet

- 1 zucchini, small
- Handful of amaranth or dandelion greens
- Handful of sprouted hemp seeds
- 1 tbs. tahini
- Sesame seeds, to taste

Directions

1. Set the Nori sheet on a cutting board, gleaming side facing down.

2. Arrange all the ingredients on the nori sheet, leaving to the right one inch broad margin of exposed nori.

3. Fold nori's sheet from the side nearest to you, roll it up and over the fillings, use both hands.

4. Sprinkle with sesame seeds and cut into thick pieces.

Grilled Zucchini Hummus Wrap

Ingredients

- 1 zucchini, ends removed and sliced
- 1 plum tomato, sliced, or cherry tomatoes, halved
- 1/4 sliced red onion
- 1 cup romaine lettuce or wild arugula
- 4 tbsp. homemade hummus (mashed garbanzo beans)
- 2 spelt flour tortillas
- 1 tbsp. grapeseed oil
- Sea salt and cayenne pepper, to taste

Directions

1. Heat a skillet to medium heat or grill.

Dr. Sebi Diet

2. In grapeseed oil, mix the sliced zucchini and sprinkle with sea salt and cayenne pepper.

3. Place tossed, sliced zucchini directly on grill and let cook for 3 minutes, flip over and cook for another 2 minutes. Set aside Zucchini.

4. Place the tortillas on the grill for around a minute, or until the grill marks are noticeable and the tortillas are fold-able.

Remove tortillas from grill and prepare wraps, 2 tablespoons of hummus, slices of zucchini, 1/2 cup greens, slices of onion and tomato.

Wrap firmly, and instantly savor.

Zucchini Bread Pancakes

Ingredients

- 2 cups spelt or kamut flour

- 2 tbsp. date sugar

- 1/4 cup mashed burro banana

- 1 cup finely shredded zucchini

- 2 cups homemade walnut milk

- 1/2 cup chopped walnuts

- 1 tbsp. grapeseed oil

Directions

1. Whisk flour in a large bowl with date sugar.

2. Mix in walnut milk and mashed banana burro. Stir until just blended, make sure the bowl's bottom is scraped so there are no dry mix pockets. Stir in shredded walnuts and Zucchini.

3. Heat the grapeseed oil over medium high heat in a griddle or skillet.

Dr. Sebi Diet

4. To make your pancakes, add batter onto the griddle. Cook on each side for 4-5 minutes.

5. Serve with a syrup of agave and enjoy!

Classic Homemade Hummus

Ingredients

- 1 cup cooked chickpeas

- 1/3 cup homemade tahini butter

- 2 tbsp. olive oil

- 2 tbsp. key lime juice

- A dash of onion powder

- Sea salt, to taste

Directions

1. Blend everything in a food processor or high-powered blender and serve.

Veggie Fajitas Tacos

Ingredients

- 1 onion

- Juice of 1/2 key lime

- 2 bell peppers

- Your choice of approved seasonings (onion powder, cayenne pepper)

- 6 corn-free tortillas (look for tortillas made with approved grains, like spelt or wild rice)

- 1 Tbsp. grapeseed oil

- Avocado

- 2-3 large portobello mushrooms

Dr. Sebi Diet

Directions

1. Remove mushroom stems, spoon gills out if necessary, and clear tops clean. Slice into approximately 1/3 "thick slices.

2. Slice the onion and bell peppers in thin slices.

3. Pour 1 Tbsp Grapeseed oil into a big size skillet on medium heat and onions and peppers. Cook for 2 minutes.

4. Mix in seasonings and mushrooms. Stir frequently, and cook for another seven-eight minutes or until tender.

5. Heat the spoon and tortillas the fajita material into the middle of the tortilla. Serve with key lime juice and avocado.

Healthy "Fried-Rice"

Ingredients

- 1 cup cooked wild rice or quinoa
- 1/2 cup sliced bell peppers
- 1/2 cup sliced mushrooms
- 1/2 cup sliced zucchini
- 1/4 onion, cubed
- 1 tbsp. grapeseed oil
- Sea salt and cayenne pepper, to taste

Directions

1. Heat oil in a pan, then sauté onion until brown.

2. Add remaining vegetables and continue to cook for another 5 minutes. Make sure they don't get too soft.

3. Add the cup of boiled rice, then simmer until lightly browned.

Dr. Sebi Diet

"Zoodles" With Avocado Sauce

Ingredients

- 2 large zucchinis

- 2 cups basil

- 1/2 cup water

- 1/2 cup walnuts

- 4 tbsp key lime juice

- 2 avocados

- 24 sliced cherry tomatoes

- Sea salt, to taste.

Directions

1. Use a peeler or Spiralizer to make the zucchini noodles.

2. Add the remaining ingredients (except the cherry tomatoes) in a blender and blend until smooth.

3. In a mixing bowl, add noodles, avocado sauce, and cherry tomatoes.

Creamy Kamut "Alkaline" Pasta

Ingredients

For Pasta

- 12 ounce spelt pasta

- 6-8 cups of spring water (to boil your pasta)

- 2 tablespoon grapeseed oil

- 1 tablespoon dried tarragon

- 1 teaspoon sea salt

- 1 teaspoon onion powder

Dr. Sebi Diet

For Creamy Sauce

- 2 tablespoon grapeseed oil, divided

- ½ medium onion, chopped

- 1/4 teaspoon black pepper plus ½ teaspoon more

- 1/4 teaspoon sea salt + plus ½ teaspoon more

- 1/4 cup chickpea flour

- 2 cups spring water

- 16 ounce sliced baby bella mushrooms

- 15-ounce full-fat unsweetened can coconut milk

- 1 tablespoon dried tarragon

- 1 teaspoon dried oregano

- 1 teaspoon dried basil

- 2 teaspoon onion powder

- 2-3 plum (roma) tomatoes, chopped

- 2 cups packed fresh kale

Directions

Pasta

1. Bring water to a boil and grab a big bowl. Add a pinch of salt to the water to taste.

2. Upon boiling water, add spelt pasta. Allow it to cook for almost 8 to 10 min until pasta is a bit firm. Once the pasta has boiled, drain and add to a bowl. (Keep out the pot because you'll use it to prepare the sauce.) 3. OPTIONAL: We'll be seasoning the pasta here individually while still hot. This step can be missed if you want. Add the grapeseed oil, dried tarragon, sea salt, and onion powder to your warm pasta.

3. Mix the pasta coating evenly with the seasonings. Take one shell of pasta and ensure you can feel the seasonings on it. Set aside your creamy sauce to start making.

Creamy Sauce

1. Add 1 tablespoon of grapeseed oil to the same large pot used to cook the pasta. Place over medium to high heat, allowing 1 minute of oil to heat up. Put in chopped onions and chopped mushrooms to the heated oil. Cook for about 3 to 5 minutes, occasionally stirring until vegetables soften.

2. Add 1/4 teaspoon salt and 1/4 teaspoon pepper to season and mix in the vegetables. Add 1 tablespoon of grapeseed oil and chickpea flour. Combine the flour with the oil and vegetables continuously for no more than 1 minute. There should be no spots of flour. That will make your sauce thicken.

3. Then, add coconut milk, dried tarragon, dried oregano, dried basil, onion powder, 1/2 tsp. of sea salt, and 1/2 tsp. of black pepper into the spring water. Stir to mix and leave to boil uncovered at low heat for around 20 minutes before the sauce starts to thicken slightly.

4. After about 20 minutes, add tomatoes and kale in your cooked pasta. Stir for around 3 to 5 minutes until kale is cooked, then remove from heat. Do not stress if, when you add your pasta, the creamy sauce becomes somewhat liquid, and not as creamy. To get the creamy feeling, the starches in the pasta can help thicken it up even further.

5. Serve alone or with Fried Oyster Mushrooms right away. One portion is around 11/2-2 cups.

6. This recipe stays fresh in the fridge for around 3-4 days.

"Alkaline" Blackberry Breakfast Bars

Ingredients

- 4 baby bananas (or 3 burro bananas)

- ½ cup grapeseed oil

- ¼ cup agave nectar

- 2 cup quinoa flakes

- 1 cup spelt flour

- ¼ teaspoon sea salt

- 1 cup Alkaline Blackberry Jam

Directions

1. Heat your oven to 350 ° F. Take a wide mixing bowl and smash baby bananas.

2. Then apply the grapeseed oil and agave nectar to the banana smash and blend well until it is thoroughly mixed.

3. Add the quinoa flakes and spelt flour into the moist mixture. Combine everything to make a sticky dough when pressed between your fingers.

4. Taking 2⁄3 of a mixture and press uniformly into a parchment pan measuring 9 x 9 inches square sheet. Next, top up with your Alkaline Blackberry Jam and spread uniformly. Round it off with the crumbling of the leftover dough mixture.

5. Bake uncovered for 20 minutes. Remove from heat until done and allow bars to cool for at least 15 minutes before cutting.

6. These bars can last about 5 or 6 days in the refrigerator, and about 3 months in the freezer.

Kamut Raisin Pancakes

Ingredients

- 2 cups of Kamut flour

- 1 glass of maple crystals

- 2 table spoon of vanilla extract

- 1 2/3 tsp of seams powder

Dr. Sebi Diet

- 1 1/2 glass of almond milk
- 1/4 cup of raisins

Directions

1. Place kamut flour, seamos powder in a bowl
2. Add raisins, vanilla extract and maple crystals
3. Mix in almond milk Put into heated pan and simmer on both sides

Kamut Puff Cereal

Ingredients

- 1/4 cup of chopped almonds
- 1 cup of hot Almond milk
- 1/4 of raisins
- 1 cup of kamut puffs
- 1/4 cup of chopped dates
- 1/4 cup of agave nectar

Directions

1. Add almond milk to Almonds, dates, agave nectar, cereals, and Enjoy.

Mushroom Patties

Ingredients

- 1 Pinch of cayenne pepper
- 1/4 bunch of cilantros
- 1/2 cup bell peppers
- 1/4 tsp oregano
- 2 tsp onion powder.
- 4 tbs sea salt

Dr. Sebi Diet

- 2 portabella mushrooms

- 1 tsp dill

- 1/4 cup of spelt flour

Directions

1. Steep mushrooms for one minute in warm water

2. Remove and put mushrooms in a food processor from bell peppers and scallions Apply flour, cilantro, and some other seasonings

3. Mix gently and shape into patties

4. Put them in a heated fry pan with two tbs of olive oil

5. Fry on every sides until cooked (about three minutes each)

The best Greens

Ingredients

- 2 cups of chopped onions

- 3 bunches of turnips greens and mustard 1/2 of each

- 1 tsp of chili powder

- 3 tbs sea salt

- 1/4 cup olive oil

Directions

1. Heat up the pan then putt onions, cook until golden.

2. Add greens and cook at least for twenty min.

3. season with cayenne or chili powder and sea salt

Vegetable Patties

Ingredients

- 2 chayote squash diced

Dr. Sebi Diet

- Kamut Flour

- 1 pinch of African red pepper

- 1 bunch of kale greens cut fine

- 1 bunch of broccolis chopped fine

- 3 tbs olive oil

- 1 medium yellow onion chopped fine

- Spring Water

- 1/4 cup sea moss powder

- 1/2 red and green peppers chopped

Directions

1. heat container with 3 tbs olive oil

2. add onion, chayote squash, bell pepper, and African red pepper

3. ground cumin, fry for 2-3 minutes

4. add kale simmer and broccoli 10-12 minutes

Kamut Flour

1. mix sea moss with enough water and flour for making a dough

2. roll out the dough on all purpose flour board and split into 10 inches diameter circles and put fried vegetables half of circle

3. fold the remaining half to protect the vegetables

4. using a fork to keep the edges closed

5. put patties on an oiled baking tray and bake twenty-thirty minutes or until light brown

Vegetable Stir Fry Medley

Ingredients

Dr. Sebi Diet

- 1 small red and green pepper, chopped

- 2 zucchinis, sliced

- 1 pkg. oyster mushrooms, sliced

- 3 tbs olive oil

- 1/2 small yellow onion, chopped fine

- 1 cup broccoli, chopped fine

- 8 cherry tomatoes, chopped

Directions

1. Put olive oil in a warm stainless-steel tray.

2. add onions and tomatoes

3. add your best toppings and cook for 3_4 min

4. add sauté and mushrooms for another 3_4 min

5. add broccoli, bell peppers, zucchini, and sauté 3_4 minutes

Vegetable & Rice Noodles

Ingredients

- 1 portion rice noodles

- 2 lettuce leaves or other greens

- 2 cups mixed vegetables

- 1/2 cube stock

- 2 cups of water

- 1/2 tsp butter (optional)

Direction

1. Put cubes in the skillet, then pour in water and let boil for 1 minute

2. Add in vegetables and let it boil for 2 mins

Dr. Sebi Diet

3. Add noodles to the pot – break apart first or use as they are. It depends on how you like to eat them

4. Stir, cover and let boil for two minutes

5. Add greens

6. Leave covered for another minute

7. Stir in butter

5.2 Salads

Dandelion Strawberry Salad

Ingredients

- 2 tbsp. grapeseed oil

- 1 medium red onion, sliced

- 10 ripe strawberries, sliced

- 2 tbsp. key lime juice

- 4 cups dandelion greens

- Sea salt to taste

Directions

1. First of all, warm grapeseed oil in a 12-inch non-stick frying pan over medium heat. Add some sliced onions and a small pinch of sea salt. Cook until the onions are soft, lightly brown, and reduced to about 1/3 of raw volume, stirring frequently.

2. Then toss strawberry slices in a tiny bowl with 1 teaspoon of key lime juice. Rinse the dandelion greens and, if you prefer, slice them into chunks of bite-size.

3. When the onions are about to be cooked, add the remaining key lime juice to the saucepan and keep on cooking until it has thickened to coat the onions for a minute or two. Remove the onions from heat.

4. Combine the vegetables, onions, and strawberries with all their juices in a salad bowl. Sprinkle with sea salt.

Headache Preventing Salad

Ingredients

- 1/2 seeded cucumber
- 2 cups watercress
- 2 tbsp. olive oil
- 1 tbsp key lime juice
- Salt and cayenne pepper, to taste.

Directions

1. Combine with the olive oil and key lime until well blended.
2. Have watercress and cucumber arranged.
3. Add the dressing to taste, then sprinkle with salt and pepper.

Detox Watercress Citrus Salad

Ingredients

- 1 avocado, ripe
- 4 cups watercress
- 1 Seville orange, zested, peeled and sliced
- 2 very thin slices red onion
- 2 tsp. agave syrup
- 2 tbsp. Key lime juice
- 2 tbsp. olive oil
- 1/8 tsp. salt
- Cayenne pepper, optional

Directions

1. Set on two plates watercress, avocado, onion and oranges.

2. In a small bowl, mix together the key lime juice, olive oil, agave syrup, salt and cayenne pepper.

3. When ready to be served, spoon the dressing over salad.

Basil Avocado Pasta Salad

Ingredients

- 1 avocado, chopped

- 1 cup fresh basil, chopped

- 1-pint cherry tomatoes halved

- 1 tbsp. key lime juice

- 1 tsp. agave syrup

- 1/4 cup olive oil

- 4 cups cooked spelt-pasta

Directions

1. Place the cooked pasta in a huge bowl.

2. Add the avocado, basil, and tomatoes and mix until completely blended.

3. Whisk the oil, lime juice, agave syrup, and sea salt together in a deep mixing pot.

Toss over the pasta, then stir to blend.

The Grilled Romaine Lettuce Salad

Ingredients

- 4 small heads romaine lettuce, rinsed

- 1 tbsp. red onion, chopped finely

- 1 tbsp. key lime juice

Dr. Sebi Diet

- Onion powder, to taste

- 1 tbsp. fresh basil, chopped

- Sea salt and cayenne pepper, to taste

- 4 tbsp. olive oil

- 1 tbsp. agave syrup

Directions

1. Place halves of lettuce in a wide non-stick pan cut side down. Do not add oil. Observe the lettuce color by turning them around. Check that the lettuce browns on both faces.

2. Take off the pan from heat and let the lettuce cool down on a broad platter.

3. In a small mixing pot, add red onion and olive oil, agave syrup, key lime juice, and fresh basil for dressing. Sprinkle with salt and cayenne pepper. Whisk to blend properly.

4. Transfer grilled lettuce and drizzle with the dressing onto a serving plate.

5. Enjoy it!

Alkaline Vegan Salad

Ingredients

- 1 small head of lettuce, cut thinly

- 1 medium-sized onion, chopped in small pieces

- 10 plum tomatoes, cut in small pieces

- Juice of 1 orange

- 1/2 cucumber, spiraled, cut in small pieces or sliced

- 1/2 apple peeled and diced

- 1/2 teaspoon cayenne pepper

Dr. Sebi Diet

- A pinch of salt

Direction

1. Put everything into a bowl and uniformly blend together. You may consume it as is or apply a homemade dressing, tahini, or hummus to the salad.

2. It is good enough to eat it alone, but it can be added to other foods as well.

Onion Avocado Salad

Ingredients

- 1 avocado diced or chopped in small pieces

- 2 medium-sized onion, sliced or diced

- 6 to 8 cherry or plum tomatoes, sliced or diced

- 1 tsp lime juice (optional)

- A pinch of sea salt (optional)

- 1/2 tsp cayenne pepper

Direction

1. In a pot, add the onion, avocado, and tomato and blend well to mix.

2. Add lime juice, sea salt, then cayenne, then toss.

You may eat this salad by itself or with vegetables, cooked quinoa, spelt dumplings, or some other alternative of your preference.

Mushroom Cucumber Salad

Ingredients

- 5 Medium-sized Mushrooms (diced)

- 2 Lettuce Leaves (chopped, thinly)

- 1/2 Cucumber (peeled and shred with a peeler to get thin slices)

- Orange Juice (juice of half of a small orange)

Dr. Sebi Diet

- 1 Tbsp Mixed Dried Herbs

- 1/4 Tsp Salt

- 2 Tbsp Lime/Lemon Juice

- 5 Cherry or Plum Tomatoes (chopped)

- 1/2 Tbsp Cayenne Pepper (or Black Pepper)

Directions

1. Combine all ingredients in a salad bowl and combine together to ensure a nice mixture of all. You can get your salad straight away or place it in the fridge for at least an hour to marinate the flavors.

Mushroom Tomato Salad

Ingredients

- 1 Small Tangerine juice

- 2 Stalks Scallion / spring onions, diced

- 6 Medium sized mushrooms, diced

- 6 Cherry or plum tomatoes, cut in quarters

- 2 Spring Coriander/ cilantro, diced

- 1/2 Medium lime or 1 small lime juice

- 1 Tsp Dried herbs

- 1 Tsp Olive oil

- 1/2 Tsp Turmeric

- 1/2 Tsp Cayenne pepper

- 1/2 Tsp Sea salt

Directions

Dr. Sebi Diet

1. In a bowl, mix mushroom, tomato, scallion, cilantro, and toss 2. Add olive oil, lime juice, dried herbs, then mix 3. Add tangerine juice and mix together

2. Let stand for an hour on counter or refrigerate for longer duration. If you choose, you may use salad dressing but this is not required. Use it as your side meal or main course.

Pasta Salad

Ingredients

- 2 boxes of spelt penne
- 2 avocados cut in small pieces
- 1/2 cup of chopped onions
- 1/4 cup of almond milk
- 1/4 cup of fresh lime juice
- 3 tbs of maple syrup
- 1 1/2 cup of sun-dried tomatoes
- 4 tbs of sea salt
- 3-4 dashes of cilantro
- 1/2 cup of olive oil

Directions

1. Cook the pasta as per the instructions
2. Add everything in a big bowl
3. Toss until evenly distributed

Easy Salad

Ingredients

- 6 lettuce leaves

Dr. Sebi Diet

- 6 cherry or plum tomatoes, chopped

- 3-4 mushrooms, chopped

- 1/2 cucumber, chopped

- 10 olives

- Juice of half of a lime

- 1 tsp coconut oil/olive oil (optional)

Directions

1. Put the lettuce in a bowl, break it with your hand into pieces. Add mushroom, sliced tomatoes, and cucumber. Mix all up together.

2. Add olives, lime juice, cold-pressed oil, and salt. Mix all up together.

3. They are ready to eat.

Salad Alkaline Electric Recipe

Ingredients

- Romaine Lettuce

- 1 Kale

- 4 Roma Tomatoes

- 1 Yellow Pepper

- 1 Orange Pepper

- 2 Red Onion

- 3 Jalapeno

- Extra Virgin Olive Oil (Apply as desired)

- Apple Cider Vinegar (Optional)

Directions

1. Rinse and dry all the ingredients

2. Chop the ingredients

3. Place them in a bowl

4. Sprinkle extra virgin olive oil (apply as desired)

Optional: Add Apple Cider Vinegar (apply as desired)

Simple Fruit Salad

Ingredients

- 1 banana

- 1 persimmon

- 1 mango

- 1 apple

- 6 – 7 dates

Directions

1. Wash and slice apple, mango then persimmon, then mix in a bowl.

2. Peel and cut banana, add with date in bowl.

Mushroom Salad

Ingredients

- 1/4 bunch fresh spinach, torn

- 1/4 bunch red leaf lettuce, torn

- 1/4 bunch romaine lettuce, torn

- 1/2 lb. fresh mushrooms

- 1/2 red bell pepper, chopped

- 1 sm. red onion, diced

- 1/2 cup olive oil

- 1/4 cup fresh lime juice

Dr. Sebi Diet

- 1/2 tsp. dill

- 1/2 tsp. basil

- 1/2 tsp. sea salt

Directions

1. Thoroughly wash mushrooms, dry, slice

2. Add onion, bell pepper, olive oil, lime juice, dill, sea salt, and basil

3. Marinade 1/2 hour in the refrigerator

4. Thoroughly wash greens, dry and shred

5. Place greens with mushrooms and mix thoroughly

6. Enjoy!

5.3 Milk Alternatives – Nut, Seed and Grain Milk

Why make your own milk?

- There will be a fresh product for you.

- You know just what's in there.

- Preservatives and chemicals are used in the market made milk. Some can also contain vitamins and minerals, which are inorganic.

- You get the natural 'real' nutrients.

- Certain supermarket brands bought only contain a limited amount of the actual milk.

- Producing your own is more cost-efficient.

- You can add something you like, including a bit of date sugar or cinnamon, in a versatile way.

- You should do it to your precise preference.

Nuts, Seeds, and Grains Used to Make Milk

Dr. Sebi Diet

Just about any nut, seed or grain can be used, including almond, brazil nut, hazelnut, cashew, pinenut, spelt, quinoa, kamut, rye, oats, wild rice, fonio, tef, coconut, and many more.

General Recipe

- 1 cup nuts, seeds or grains

- 3 cups of filtered water

- 3 tbsp. sweetener (coconut sugar, agave, date sugar or 3-4 pitted dates)

- 1 tbsp coconut butter (optional)

- 1 teaspoon natural vanilla (optional)

- Pinch of sea salt (optional)

Directions

1. Soak the seeds, nuts, or grains for at least 6 hours or longer.

2. Drain grains, nuts or seeds and then wash.

3. Add 3 cups of water to mixer. Mix in remaining ingredients and blend until smooth.

4. Strain with a nut milk bag, strainer or cheese cloth (Some nut milks do not need strain due to smoothness, but test the mixture and see if you're Fine with it as it is).

5. Serve cold, or warm at room temperature, or add as needed to certain recipes and dishes.

Note: Place in fridge in a container. This milk won't last as long as the market purchased milk, so it will be better to use it for future usage within two or three days or freeze.

Amaranth Milk

Ingredients

Dr. Sebi Diet

- 1/2 cup raw amaranth
- 2 cups filtered water

Directions

1. Steep in water for 6 to 12 hours or toast for 5 minutes in oven at 350 F. Rinse the amaranth soaked through a cheesecloth, because they are very small. Shake with water, then filter via a bag of nut milk or cheese cloth.

Brazil Nuts Milk

Ingredients

- 1/2 cup raw Brazil nuts
- 2 cups filtered water

Directions

1. Steep in water for 6 to 12 hours or toast for 5 minutes in oven at 350 F. Rinse the amaranth soaked through a cheesecloth, because they are very small. Shake with water, then filter via a bag of nut milk or cheese cloth.

Hazelnuts Milk

Ingredients

- 1/2 cup raw hazelnuts
- 2 cups filtered water

Directions

1. Steep in water for 6 to 12 hours or toast for 5 minutes in oven at 350 F. Rinse the amaranth soaked through a cheesecloth, because they are very small. Shake with water, then filter via a bag of nut milk or cheese cloth.

Pine Nuts Milk

Ingredients

- 1 cup raw pine nuts

Dr. Sebi Diet

- 3 cups filtered water

- 1 teaspoon vanilla (optional)

- 1/4 teaspoon salt

- 1 tablespoon date sugar or agave (optional)

Directions

1. Steep in water for 6 to 12 hours or toast for 5 minutes in oven at 350 F. Rinse the amaranth soaked through a cheesecloth, because they are very small. Shake with water, then filter via a bag of nut milk or cheese cloth.

Hemp Seeds Milk

Ingredients

- 1 1/2 cups hemp seeds

- 2 1/2 cups filtered water

Directions

1. Steep in water for 6 to 12 hours or toast for 5 minutes in oven at 350 F. Rinse the amaranth soaked through a cheesecloth, because they are very small. Shake with water, then filter via a bag of nut milk or cheese cloth.

Quinoa Milk

Ingredients

- 1 cup quinoa (rinsed and cooked)

- 1 tablespoon date sugar or agave (optional)

- 2 cups filtered water, and up to 6 cups of water

- 1 teaspoon vanilla extract (optional)

Directions

Dr. Sebi Diet

1. Steep in water for 6 to 12 hours or toast for 5 minutes in oven at 350 F. Rinse the amaranth soaked through a cheesecloth, because they are very small. Shake with water, then filter via a bag of nut milk or cheese cloth.

Sesame Milk

Ingredients

- 1 cup raw sesame seeds (ground)

- 2 cups filtered water

- 1 tablespoon date sugar or agave (optional)

Directions

1. Steep in water for 6 to 12 hours or toast for 5 minutes in oven at 350 F. Rinse the amaranth soaked through a cheesecloth, because they are very small. Shake with water, then filter via a bag of nut milk or cheese cloth.

Spelt Milk

Ingredients

- 1 cup rolled spelt

- 3 cups filtered water

Directions

1. Steep in water for 6 to 12 hours or toast for 5 minutes in oven at 350 F. Rinse the amaranth soaked through a cheesecloth, because they are very small. Shake with water, then filter via a bag of nut milk or cheese cloth.

Kamut Milk

Ingredients

- 1 cup rolled kamut

- 3 cups filtered water

Directions

Dr. Sebi Diet

1. Steep in water for 6 to 12 hours or toast for 5 minutes in oven at 350 F. Rinse the amaranth soaked through a cheesecloth, because they are very small. Shake with water, then filter via a bag of nut milk or cheese cloth.

Wild Rice Milk

Ingredients

- 1/4 cup uncooked wild rice

- 1 cup of cooked

- 3 cups filtered water

- 3 soaked dates (optional)

Directions

1. Steep in water for 6 to 12 hours or toast for 5 minutes in oven at 350 F. Rinse the amaranth soaked through a cheesecloth, because they are very small. Shake with water, then filter via a bag of nut milk or cheese cloth.

Chickpea Milk

Ingredients

- 2-3 cups of chickpeas (garbanzo beans)

- Filtered water

- 2 to 3 tablespoon date sugar or agave (to taste, optional)

- 1/2 teaspoon sea salt (to taste)

Directions

1. Steep in water for 6 to 12 hours or toast for 5 minutes in oven at 350 F. Rinse the amaranth soaked through a cheesecloth, because they are very small. Shake with water, then filter via a bag of nut milk or cheese cloth.

2. Put on a medium-heat pot with water on the stove, add chickpea paste and let it boil for around 20 minutes. Let it cool, then strain.

Dr. Sebi Diet

Oat Milk

Ingredients

- 1 cup steel-cut oats
- 4 cups filtered water
- 1 1/2 tablespoon date sugar or agave (optional)
- 1/2 teaspoon vanilla (optional)
- 1/4 teaspoon fine grain sea salt

Directions

1. Mix the oats with warm water about 4 cups, then cool overnight.
2. Mix in with water and strain.

Coconut Milk

Ingredients

- 2 mature coconuts
- 4 cups filtered water (preferably warm)

Directions

1. Remove coconut off the shell. You can opt to remove the outer brown portion. Split into smaller bits.
2. Mix in with water and strain.

Chia Walnut Milk Recipe

Ingredients

- 4 tablespoon chia seeds
- 2 tablespoon raw walnuts
- 2 tablespoon raw sesame tahini
- 2 tablespoon date sugar or agave

Dr. Sebi Diet

- 1 teaspoon vanilla extract

- 5 cups filtered water

Directions

1. Soak seeds and walnuts in 3 cups of water overnight. Put into blender, add 1 cup of water and process at medium level. Pour in tahini, date sugar or agave and vanilla, then add 1 more cup of water. Mix until smooth.

5.4 Soups

Cucumber Basil Gazpacho

Ingredients

- 1 perfectly ripe avocado

- 1 seeded cucumber: skin left on, seeds removed

- 2 small handfuls fresh basil

- 2 cups water

- 1 1/4 teaspoon sea salt

- Juice of 1 key lime

Directions

1. Both products will be refrigerated until cold.

2. Put cooled ingredients in a blender and purée until smooth, allowing for a few specks of green to linger all over.

3. Transfer the soup to the fridge, and cool until ready to eat.

4. Garnish with rings of finely sliced cucumber and basil leaves.

Roasted Tomato and Bell Pepper Soup

Ingredients

- 4 ripe Roma tomatoes

Dr. Sebi Diet

- 3 red bell peppers

- 3 sprigs fresh thyme

- 1/4 cup homemade vegetable broth

- Pure sea salt, to taste

- Sesame oil

Directions

1. Preheat oven to 375 F.

2. Chop peppers into quarters and remove centers.

3. Slice tomatoes and put bell peppers onto a rimmed baking sheet.

4. Sprinkle with sesame oil generously, then sprinkle with sea salt.

5. Disperse thyme over the vegetables.

6. Roast it for 35-40 minutes in a preheated oven.

7. Transfer all to a food processor or blender.

8. Add heated puree and broth until smooth, adding more broth to achieve desired consistency if required.

9. Sea salt is used to taste. Pour in pots, then serve hot.

Chickpea Soup

Ingredients

- 2 cups of chickpeas

- 1 small zucchini

- 1 bell pepper

- 1 small onion

- Water

- Seasoning of your choice

Dr. Sebi Diet

Directions

1. Put all ingredients in a pot and cook over medium heat until the vegetables are aldente.

2. Once the vegetables and the soup are ready, take a multi-quick hand blender and combine well. This way, it is simplest and enjoyable. That will make ample soup for a few days.

Alkaline Electric Soup

Ingredients

- 1-2 cups of Kamut Pasta/Approved Pasta

- 1/2 cup Quinoa (Optional)

- 1 Zucchini Squash, chopped

- 2 Roma Tomatoes, diced

- 2 cups Butternut Squash, chopped

- 1/2 lb. Garbanzo Beans (cooked)*

- 1/2 cup of chopped Red Peppers

- 2 cups Mushrooms, chopped

- 1/2 cup of chopped Green Peppers

- 1 Small Red Onion, chopped

- 1/2 Gallon Spring Water (use as per need)

- 1 tsp. Dill

- 1 tsp Red Cayenne Pepper

- 1 tbsp. of Grapeseed Oil

- 1 tsp. Oregano

- 1 tbsp. Sea Salt

- 1 tsp. Basil

*Leave the garbanzo beans in water overnight and cook them prior to adding the beans to the Stew.

Directions

1. Pour the water into a wide bowl, and turn to medium heat.

2. Chop all the veggies.

3. Add the ingredients (including seasonings) to the pot and bring to a simmer for about 1 hour.

4. Stir for every 15 minutes.

5. Enjoy it!

You can freeze the remaining stew another day!

Greens Soup Recipe

Ingredients

- 2 cups leafy greens

- 1 small zucchini

- 1 bell pepper

- 1 small onion

- Water

- Seasoning of your choice

Directions

1. Put everything in a pot and cook over medium heat until the vegetables are semi-hard. Switch off the burner, let it cool off, and mix properly.

Vegetable Mushroom Soup

Ingredients

Dr. Sebi Diet

- 1 lb oyster mushrooms, chopped

- 1 bunch spinach, washed and steamed

- 1 cup quinoa

- 1 small green and red bell pepper chopped

- 2 tbs olive oil

- 1/2 lb kamut spiral pasta

- 2 onions chopped finely

- 2 large chayote squash, peeled and chopped

- 2-3 bunches kale

- Springwater

- 1 clove

- 1/2 tsp: marjoram, oregano, rosemary, thyme, red pepper, and cumin

Directions

1. put olive oil in heated skillet

2. sauté mushrooms, onions and bell peppers slowly for 20 minutes then add the mushroom mixture in the soup pot and fill with spring water

3. then add chayote squash

4. add thyme, marjoram, rosemary, oregano, red pepper, clove, cumin, and quinoa

5. Cook for 45 minutes

6. add Kamut Pasta and simmer for another 15 min

7. add spinach, mix, and then serve when tender

5.5 Desserts

Sea Moss Blueberries Pudding

Ingredients

Dr. Sebi Diet

- 3 tablespoons of sea moss gel

- 1 handful blueberries

- 1 medium/large ripe banana

- 1/4 cup or more Water

Directions

1. Add all the ingredients to a processor, along with water, and process until smooth. Begin with only 1/4 cup of water and add more if required based on the thickness of the pudding you like.

2. Enjoy it or drink chilled.

Banana Flax Chia Pudding

Ingredients

- 2 Bananas

- 1 Apple

- 2 Tbsp Flaxseed

- 1 Tbsp Chia seed

- 1 Cup Water

- 2 Tbsp Frozen Berries or Topping of choice

Directions

1. Add the bananas and apple with the water processor and combine 2. Add the mixture of flaxseed and chia seed, and blend until smooth 3. Pour in a pot, and garnish as needed.

Alkaline Electric Date Sugar

This recipe will make about 1 1/2 cups of Date Sugar.

Ingredients

- Around 8 oz. Dates

- Blender
- Food Processor
- Baking Sheet

You can use the seed dates or pitted dates in them. If the dates you use are large, more baking time can be needed.

Directions

1. Preheat Oven to 400 ° F 2. Cut the dates in half and take the seeds out. (What a sticky step!) 3. Place the dates on the sheet to cook.

2. Bake for around 12 to 15 minutes, when cooked, the dates should look slightly burnt so as long as you don't overcook them, you're going to be perfect.

3. Once the baking of dates is done, let them cool down completely.

4. They should be as hard as a candy after the dates have cooled. (Bake them for around 3-5 more minutes, if the dates are not hard).

5. Grind them up for 10 seconds in the blender.

6. Enjoy your Alkaline Date Sugar!

Alkaline Electric Brazil Nut Cheesecake

Ingredients

Cheesecake Mixture:

- 2 cups Brazil Nuts
- 1 1/2 cups Hemp Milk or Walnut Milk
- 1/4 cup Agave
- 5-6 Dates
- 2 tbsp. lime Juice
- 1 tbsp. Sea Moss Gel
- 1/4 tsp. Sea Salt

Crust:

- 1 1/2 cups Dates
- 1 1/2 cups Coconut Flakes
- 1/4 cup Agave
- 1/4 tsp. Sea Salt

Toppings:

- Mango, sliced
- Strawberries, sliced
- Raspberries, sliced
- Blueberries
- Blackberries

Tools:

- Food Processor
- Blender
- 8-inch spring form Pan
- Parchment Paper

Directions

1. Place all ingredients of the crust into a food processor and mix for 20 seconds.
2. Spread crust into a spring pan lined with parchment paper.
3. Place thinly sliced mango in a freezer along the corners of the pan.
4. Add all ingredients from the cheesecake mixture to blend and mix until smooth.
5. Pour the mixture onto the crust, cover it with foil and allow 3-4 hours to set.
6. Remove the form pan, layer with your toppings and enjoy!

Make sure the leftovers are kept in the fridge.

Berry Sorbet

Ingredients

- 1/2 cup date sugar

Dr. Sebi Diet

- 1 1/2 tsp. spelt flour

- 2 cups strawberries (pureed)

- 2 cups water

Directions

1. In a broad pan, dissolve the date sugar and flour in the water over low heat, then simmer for around ten minutes until thick, like syrup. Remove from heat and refrigerate.

2. Add the pureed fruit when the syrup is fully cooled, and blend properly.

3. Split the sorbet into chunks, then pulse it in a blender or food processor until it is creamy and smooth.

4. Place in an uncovered plastic container and freeze until firm.

5. Place the sorbet back into the freezer and allow for a further 4 hours to freeze.

"Alkaline" Vegan Blackberry Jam

Ingredients

- 3 six-ounce package fresh blackberries

- 3 tablespoons agave nectar

- 1 tablespoon squeezed key lime juice

- ¼ cup sea moss gel + 2 tablespoons additional

Directions

1. Rinse blackberries. Then take a medium-sized pot and put on medium-high heat. Stir up the blackberries once the berries start releasing liquid.

2. Upon the breakdown of the blackberries, take your immersion blender to break down the remaining large chunks. NOTE: To break down the berries, you can use a potato masher or fork. Or extract them from the pot and mix to render them smooth in your blender or food processor.

3. Add the agave nectar, key lime juice, and sea moss gel next. Whisk over medium-low flame for 1 to 2 minutes before the jam begins to thicken. The gel of sea moss will thicken the jam relatively easily.

4. Remove from heat, and allow for 15 minutes to cool.

5. Use with cookies, pancakes, waffles (or something else that you'd usually have jam on).

6. Move on to a new sterile mason jar unless immediately used. Make sure the lid is tightly closed—store for 5-7 days in the refrigerator or for 2 months in the freezer.

Blueberry Spelt Muffins

Ingredients

- 1/4 tsp of sea salt

- 1/3 cup of maple syrup

- 1 tsp of baking powder

- 1/2 cup of sea moss

- 1/2 cup of sea moss

- 3/4 cup of spelt flour

- 1 cup of almond milk

- 3/4 cup of kamut flour

- 1 cup of blueberries

Directions

1. Preheat Oven to 400F.

2. Put the baking cups in a muffin tray. In a mixing bowl, add flour, syrup, salt, baking powder, and sea moss.

3. Stir in almond milk. Mix in blueberries Pour in baking cups and bake for 25-30 minutes

Spelt French Toast

Ingredients

- 2 slices of Spelt Bread

- 1 cup of Almond Milk

- 2 tsp of Quinoa flakes

- 2 tsp of spelt flour

- 2 tsp of maple crystals

- 1/2 tsp of sea salt

Directions

1. Mix all ingredients together

2. Dip bread till soaking but not soggy.

3. Apply oil to the saucepan and cook gently on both sides

Xave's Delight

Ingredients

- 2 fresh limes squeezed

- 3 tbs. maple syrup

- 3 oz. sesame tahini

- 1 oz spring water

- 1 tsp. sea salt

- 1/2 tsp. red pepper

Directions

1. Add the juice of 2 limes, maple syrup, water, sea salt in a glass bottle

Dr. Sebi Diet

2. red pepper, and sesame tahini

3. Shake well and dress your salad!!

Alkaline Blueberry Spelt Pancakes

Ingredients

- 2 cups of Spelt Flour
- 1 cup of Milk (Coconut)
- 1/2 cup of Alkaline or Spring Water
- 2 Tbsp. of Grapeseed Oil
- 1/2 Cup of Agave
- 1/2 Cup of Blueberries
- 1/4 Tsp. of Sea Mose

Directions

1. In a large bowl, combine your spelt flour, hemp seeds, sea moose, agave, and grapeseed oil. (It is vital that you do NOT add hemp milk now as it can produce lumps until the grapeseed oil is in contact)

2. Mix the hemp milk in 1 cup and add the spring water until you have the consistency you want.

3. Stuff the batter onto the blueberries.

4. Heat your skillet to medium heat and use grapeseed oil to coat it lightly.

5. Pour the batter into the skillet and allow to cook on each side for around 3-5 minutes.

6. Enjoy your Pancakes Blueberry Spelt!

Alkaline Blueberry Muffins

Ingredients

- 1 cup of Coconut Milk
- 3/4 cup of Spelt Flour

Dr. Sebi Diet

- 3/4 Teff Flour
- 1/2 cup of Blueberries
- 1/3 cup of Agave
- 1/4 cup of Sea Moss Gel
- 1/2 tsp. Sea salt
- Grapeseed Oil

Directions

1. Preheat oven to 365 degrees 2. Grease 6 cups of standard-size muffin or line with muffin liners.

2. In a wide bowl, add coconut milk, flour, agave, sea salt, and sea moss gel until fully combined, then fold in blueberries.

3. Coat lightly with grape seed oil on muffin pan and dump in muffin batter.

4. Bake 30 minutes, until it reaches golden brown and springy.

5.6 Shakes, Smoothies, Juices

Sea moss Breakfast Shake

Ingredients

- 4 tbsp of almond butter
- 1 cup of maple syrup
- 3 cups of almond milk
- 3 tsp of vanilla extract
- 2 tsp of cinnamon
- 1 tsp of sea moss
- 3-4 cups of water

Direction

1. Blend hot water and sea moss.

Dr. Sebi Diet

2. Add almond butter, cinnamon, maple syrup, vanilla extract, and almond milk.

3. Blend until smooth and serve

Alkaline Electric Ginger Shot

Makes 2 shots

Ingredients

- 2 ounces of fresh ginger root
- 1 medium apple
- juice extractor or blender
- cheese cloth (optional)

Directions

1. Using a Peeler or Spoon to Remove skin from ginger

2. Chop and add to extractor.

3. Cut the apple and add ginger juice of Juice

4. Add chopped ginger & apple to mixer if using a blender.

5. Add 1-2 cups of spring water

6. Mix well

7. Filter via cheese cloth

8. Enjoy the drink

Alkaline Electric Limeade

This recipe will yield 2 1/2 cups to 3 cups of limeade.

Ingredients

- Key Limes/Limes
- Blue Agave
- Spring Water
- Ice

- Strawberries
- Blender

Directions

1. Process all the components in the blender and serve cold.

Alkaline Frozen Strawberry Limeade

Ingredients

- 1 cup Spring Water
- 1/4 cup of Lime Juice
- 1/4 cup Agave
- 1/2 cup Strawberries
- 6-8 Ice Cubes

Directions

1. Cut the leaves off, then halve the strawberries.

2. In blender add all ingredients.

3. Blend in for 10 seconds or until you hear the ice.

4. Enjoy the Frozen Strawberry Limeade in Alkaline!

Alkaline Limeade

Ingredients

- 2 cups Spring Water
- 1/4 cup of Lime Juice
- 1/4 cup of Agave

Directions

1. Drop all of the ingredients into a processor.

2. Blend in for 10 seconds together.

3. Serve with ice, or let it cool in refrigerator.

Dr. Sebi Diet

4. Have fun drinking your Alkaline Limeade!

Orange Creamsicle Smoothie

Ingredients

- 3 Seville oranges, peeled
- 1/2 Burro banana
- 1 cup coconut water
- Date sugar, to taste
- 1/2 tsp. Bromide Plus Powder

Directions

1. Add all the components to your blender and blend until smooth. Serve and enjoy!

Green Detox Smoothie

Ingredients

- 1/2 burro banana
- 1 cup Romaine lettuce
- 2 – 3 tbsp. key lime juice
- 1/2 cup ginger tea
- 1/4 cup blueberries
- 1/2 cup soft jelly coconut water

Directions

1. Prepare your tea, and let it cool.
2. Mix together all the ingredients, and enjoy!

Iron Power Smoothie

Ingredients

- 1/2 large red apple
- 1 tbsp. currants or raisins

Dr. Sebi Diet

- 1 fig
- 1/2 cup cooked quinoa
- 1 cup homemade hemp seed milk
- 2 handfuls amaranth greens
- 1 tbsp. date sugar
- 1 tsp. Bromide Plus Powder

Directions

1. Process everything in a high-powered blender until smooth and enjoy!

Sweet Sunrise Smoothie

Ingredients

- 1 cup raspberries
- 1 Seville orange
- 1/2 burro banana
- 1 cup mango
- 1 cup water

Directions

1. Process everything in a high-powered blender until smooth and enjoy!

"Stomach Soother" Smoothie

Ingredients

- 1 burro banana
- 1/2 cup prepared Dr. Sebi's Stomach Relief Herbal Tea
- 1/2 cup ginger tea
- 1 tbsp. agave syrup

Instructions

1. Prepare tea as instructed and let cool. Blend with the remaining ingredients and enjoy!

Dr. Sebi Diet

"Tropical Breeze" Smoothie

Ingredients

- 1/2 mango
- 1/2 cup cantaloupe
- 1/2 cup watermelon
- 1/2 burro banana
- 1 cup soft jelly coconut water
- 1 handful amaranth greens

Directions

1. Blend all ingredients until smooth and enjoy!

Energizer Smoothie

Ingredients

- 1 cup cubed papaya or melon
- 1 cup homemade hemp milk
- 1/2 cup cooked quinoa or amaranth
- 1 date or 1 tbsp. date sugar
- 1 tsp. Bromide Plus Powder

Directions

1. Blend all the ingredients and enjoy!

"Veggie-Ful" Smoothie

Ingredients

- 1 pear, cored and seeded
- 1/4 avocado
- 1/2 seeded cucumber, peeled
- 1 handful watercress
- 1 handful Romaine lettuce

Dr. Sebi Diet

- 1/2 cup spring water
- Date sugar, to taste (optional)

Directions

1. Process everything in a high-powered blender until smooth. Enjoy!

"Apple Pie" Smoothie

Ingredients

- 1/2 large apple
- 2 figs
- Small handful walnuts
- 1 cup ginger tea
- 1 tbsp. date sugar
- 1 tsp. Bromide Plus Powder

Directions

1. Prepare the tea and allow to cool.
2. Blend all the remaining ingredients and enjoy!

Detox Smoothie

Ingredients

- 1/2 burro banana
- 1 cup Romaine lettuce
- 2 – 3 tbsp. key lime juice
- 1/2 cup ginger tea
- 1/4 cup blueberries
- 1/2 cup soft jelly coconut water

Directions

Dr. Sebi Diet

1. Prepare tea and allow to cool.

2. Blend all ingredients together and enjoy!

Chamomile Delight Smoothie

Ingredients

- 1 burro banana

- 1/4 cup prepared Dr. Sebi's Nerve/Stress Relief Herbal Tea

- 1/2 cup homemade walnut milk

- 1 tbsp. date sugar

Directions

1. Wait for the tea to cool.

2. Blend with the left over ingredients and enjoy!

Super Hydrating Smoothie

Ingredients

- 1 cup strawberries

- 1 cup watermelon chunks

- 1 cup soft jelly coconut water

- 1 tbsp. date sugar

Directions

1. Blend all ingredients and enjoy!

Simply Delicious Vegan Berries Smoothie

Ingredients

- 2 Bananas cut into slices and frozen

- 1 handful black currants

- 1 handful red currants

Dr. Sebi Diet

- 1 handful blackberries

Direction

1. Combine everything in a blender, then blend with water. You can often use nut-milk or coconut water instead of water.

2. Serve in a glass or bowl.

3. (Optional) Decorate with berries and raisins.

Vegan Banana Ice Cream Smoothie

Ingredients

- 2 Bananas, sliced and frozen
- 1 Handful Raisins (Soaked in water for at least 2 hours)
- 1 Tablespoon Nut Butter
- 1 Cup Water (or Nut Milk)
- 1/2 Teaspoon Mixed Spice

Direction

1. Put all in a blender, and mix until smooth. Depending on how thick or thin you like it to be you may add more water or less water.

2. To thicken a little bit more, serve as is or place in a freezer.

Delicious Prickly Pear Banana Smoothie

Ingredients

- 1 Cup Prickly Pear Juice*
- 2 Ripe Bananas
- 1/2 Cup Water
- 1/2 Tsp Mixed Spices

*Blend 2 Prickly Pears with 1 Cup water, strain. It could also be ran through a juicer, this will mean you have less liquid to work with, resulting in a thicker smoothie.

Directions

1. Add everything to a mixer and blend until smooth. Pour into a glass or a small mug.

Banana Apple Flax Smoothie

Ingredients

- 2 Medium Sized Bananas
- 1/2 Apple
- 1 Tablespoon Flaxseed (ground or whole)
- 1 Cup Water

Directions

1. Mix everything in a mixer until smooth.
2. Pour in a bowl, and add favorite garnish

Valentine's Day Smoothie

Ingredients

- 1 handful frozen fruits (berries)
- 1 small apple
- 1 large banana

Directions

1. Blend and strain the berries for seed extraction.
2. Stir in chopped apple and mix.
3. Mix in banana and blend until smooth.

Green Vegetables Berry Smoothie

Ingredients

- 1 Ripe Banana
- 1 Handful of Berries
- 2 Cups of Spring Greens / Kale
- 1 Cup Water (according to the consistency you want for your smoothie. Start with 1 cup).

Direction

1. Blend everything in a mixer until smooth. Put more water, depending on the consistency of smoothie you want.

2. Instead of water, coconut water or coconut milk could also be used-that of course brings a much more flavor to the smoothie.

Apple Asparagus

Ingredients

- 2 apples
- 7 spears asparagus
- 1 small lime (Peeled)

2. Cucumber Lime

Ingredients

- 1 large cucumber
- 2 key limes

3. Orange Blueberry Ginger

Ingredients

- 4 oranges
- 1 cup blueberries

Dr. Sebi Diet

- 1 small knuckle ginger

4. Orange Canta-Kale

Ingredients

- 2 large oranges
- 1/4 cantaloupe
- 2 kale leaves

5. Greens Apple Ginger

Ingredients

- 4 large kale leaves
- 1 apple
- 1 knuckle ginger

6. Apple Ginger

Ingredients

- 3 apples
- 1 knuckle ginger

7. Kale Mango Orange

Ingredients

- 7 leaves kale
- 1 mango
- 1 orange

8. Kale Grape

Ingredients

- 1 bunch kale
- 3 cups grapes

Dr. Sebi Diet

9. Apple Strawberry

Ingredients

- 3 apples
- 8 strawberries

10. Apple Kale

Ingredients

- 1 bunch kale
- 2 apples
- 1 knuckle ginger

11. Apple Pear

Ingredients

- 1 apple
- 1 pear
- 1 small handful of dill

12. Kale Orange

Ingredients

- 6 kale leaves
- 2 oranges

13. Kale Apple Plum

Ingredients

- 3 Leaves Kale
- 1 Apple
- 2 Red Plums

14. Kale Pear

Dr. Sebi Diet

Ingredients

- 1 bunch kale
- 1 pear
- 16 oz strawberries
- 1 knuckle ginger

15. Basil Pear Mix

Ingredients

- 1 bunch kale
- 1 pear
- 1 apple
- 1 handful of basil

16. Cucumber Fresh

Ingredients

- 1/2 bunch kale (7 leaves)
- 1 large handful basil
- 1 cucumber
- 2 stalks fennel (bulb part leaves included)
- 1 knuckle ginger

17. Greens Pepper Squash

Ingredients

- 3 leaves kale
- 1 red bell pepper
- 1 yellow squash
- 1 cucumber

18. Honeydew Mix

Ingredients

- 5 leaves kale
- 2 apples
- 1/3 of a honeydew melon

19. Minty Fresh

Ingredients

- 1 head of romaine lettuce
- 1 small handful of mint
- 3 swiss chard leaves
- 1 lemon
- 1 apple

20. Green Orange Mint

Ingredients

- 4 oranges
- 6 kale leaves
- 1 small handful of mint

21. Celery Citrus Vege

Ingredients

- 1 orange
- 1/2 cucumber
- 3 celery stalks
- 1/2 lemon
- 1 fuji apple

Dr. Sebi Diet

22. Pineapple Greens

Ingredients

- 2 handfuls of spinach
- 4 kale leaves
- 1 cup pineapple
- 1 small handful of mint leaves
- 2 granny smith apples (green)

23. Zesty

Ingredients

- 1 cup fresh basil leaves
- 1 large cucumber
- 1 lime
- 1 green apple

24. Minty Kale

Ingredients

- 5 large kale leaves
- 1 lemon
- 1 large apple
- 1 knuckle ginger
- 1 sprig of fresh mint

25. Cucumber Basil

Ingredients

- 1 handful of basil leaves
- 1 cucumber

- 1/2 lime

- 1 apple, cut into wedges

26. Pine Beet

Ingredients

- 1 cup kale

- 2 Swiss chard leaves

- 1/2 cup parsley

- 1/2 small beet

- 1/2 cup pineapple

- 2 apples

- 1 sprig fresh mint

- 1/2 lemon

27. Parsley Plus

Ingredients

- 2 cups kale

- 2 green apples

- 1/2 cup parsley leaves

- 1 medium cucumber

- 2 celery stalks

- 1 (1-inch) piece of ginger

- 2 tablespoons lemon juice

28. Bitter Fresh

Ingredients

- 2 medium to large bitter melons

Dr. Sebi Diet

- 1 romaine lettuce head

- 1 large Fuji apple

- 1/2 lemon

- 1 medium cucumber

29. Tasty Bitters

Ingredients

- 2 large bitter melons

- 1 bunch of parsley

- 1 medium-sized zucchini

- 1 red apple

- 1/2 lemon

30. Greens

Ingredients

- 5 stalks celery

- 4 kale leaves

- 3 cups spinach

- 1 cucumber

- 1/2 bunch parsley

Direction for above mentioned juice

1. Blend everything in a blender until smooth. Add more water, based on how dense a smoothie you like.

Chicory Coffee

Ingredients

- 1 Tablespoon Chicory Root (roasted and grounded)

Dr. Sebi Diet

- 1 Tablespoon Dandelion root (roasted and grounded)

- 2 Cups Water

Directions

1. Place the water, root chicory, and root dandelion in a pan.

2. Bring to a boil and allow to cook for 2-3 minutes.

3. Strain with a fine-mesh strainer and serve.

Herbal Root Coffee

Ingredients

- 2 Tablespoons Dandelion Root (roasted and ground)

- 2 Tablespoons Chicory Root (roasted and ground)

- ½ Tablespoon Cinnamon Powder (optional)

- 4 Cups Water

- Natural Sweetener date sugar or agave (to taste)

Directions

1. Add the dandelion root, chicory root, cinnamon, and water to your French press or coffee machine.

2. Add the boiling water and let it steep the herbs for 5-7 minutes.

3. Strain and add a sweetener to taste (date sugar or agave).

4. Dust with cinnamon and drink.

Dandelion Chicory Carob Maca Coffee Combo

Ingredients

- 1 Tablespoon Dandelion Root (roasted and grounded)

- 1 Tablespoon Chicory Root (roasted and grounded)

- 1 Teaspoon Carob (roasted and grounded)

Dr. Sebi Diet

- 1 Teaspoon Maca Powder

- 3 Cups Water

Directions

1. Load a coffee maker with water, dandelion root, chicory root, carob, and maca powder.

2. Add boiling water, and allow for 5-7 minutes to steep.

3. Stir in sweetener to taste and drink (date sugar or agave).

Reishi Dandelion Maca Latte

Ingredients

- 4-8 Oz Coconut Milk (or any other plant-based milk of choice)

- 4 Oz Freshly Brewed Reishi Roast (steeped for 15 minutes)

- 1 Teaspoon date sugar or agave (optional)

- 1 Teaspoon Maca Powder

Directions

1. In coconut milk, heat Maca Powder only before steam arises.

2. Put into a cup and add the Reishi Roast.

3. Stir in the sweetener to taste and drink (date sugar or agave).

Dandelion Root Coffee

Ingredients

- 2 Tablespoons Dandelion Root (ground and roasted)

- 2 Tablespoons Chicory Root (ground and roasted)

- 1 Cinnamon Stick (optional)

- 4 Cups Water

Directions

Dr. Sebi Diet

1. Put water, root dandelion, root chicory, and the stick of cinnamon in a pan.

2. Allow to boil, then simmer for 5-7 minutes.

3. Strain with a fine-mesh strainer.

4. Pour into cup.

5. If needed, add coconut milk and serve.

Herbal Coffee

Ingredients

- 1 Tbsp. Pau D'Arco Powder

- 4 Tsp. Dandelion Root (roasted and grounded)

- 1 1/2 Tsp. Chicory (roasted and grounded)

- 1 Tsp. Cacao Nibs

- 4 Cups boiling water

Directions

For the roasted cacao nibs

1. Preheat oven to 350 degrees. On a small baking sheet, spread the chopped cacao nibs (1/2 cup cacao nibs, finely chopped) out.

2. Bake and remove from the oven after 5 minutes.

3. Cool and put in a container for later use.

For the herbal coffee

1. Add ingredients to a French Press or Coffee machine. Enfold with boiling water and let brew for five to seven minutes.

2. Push the filter down, then pour into a cup.

Chicory Cacao Blend

Ingredients

Dr. Sebi Diet

- 1 Cup Hot Almond Milk

- 1 Tablespoon Chicory Root (roasted and grounded)

- 1 Tablespoon Cacao Powder (roasted and grounded)

- 1 Teaspoon date sugar or agave (optional)

Directions

1. Heat 1 cup of almond milk until it is steamed and hot but does not boil.

2. Stir in chicory powder and cacao powder.

3. Stir and add sweetener.

4. Pour into a cup then serve.

Chicory Cafe Au Lait

Ingredients

- 1 Teaspoon Chicory Root (grounded and roasted)

- Plant-based Milk (Almond, Coconut, etc.)

- Water

Directions

1. In a coffee maker, add roasted chicory root and brew with water.

2. Warm the desired milk, just don't let it boil.

3. Add the milk and whisk in coffee.

4. Note: Additional roots can be added, or water can be added to make stronger coffee.

5. All the recipes, if you choose, can be rendered in a saucepan.

6. You may use your chosen plant-based milk.

Seamoss Breakfast Shake

Ingredients

Dr. Sebi Diet

- 4 tbsp. of almond butter

- 1 cup of maple syrup

- 3 cups of almond milk

- 3 tsp of vanilla extract

- 2 tsp of cinnamon

- 1 tsp of seamoss

- 3-4 cups of water

Directions

1. Blend hot water and seamoss

2. Add almond butter, maple syrup, vanilla, cinnamon extract and almond milk

3. Blend until smooth and drink

Papaya Breakfast Shake

Ingredients

- 2 cups of almond milk

- 1/2 cup of agave nectar

- 1 tsp of sea moss

- 1/2 cup of frozen or fresh papaya

- 1/2 cup of cold water

Directions

1. Blend water and sea moss together

2. Add Papaya, milk, and agave nectar

3. Blend till smooth and serve

Dr. Sebi Diet

5.7 Sauces, Dips, Dressings, Creams, Butter and Cheese

Avocado Pizza Sauce

Ingredients

- 1 Avocado
- 2 Tbsp. Chopped Onion
- 1/2 tsp. Powdered onion
- 1/2 tsp. Sea Salt
- 1/2 tsp. Oregano
- Basil (Pinch)

Directions:

1. Cut down the center of the avocado, cut the pit and scrap the insides into your food processor.

2. Add left over ingredients to the blender and blend for 3 minutes or until smooth, scraping the processor inside if necessary.

Tomato Pizza Sauce

Ingredients

- 5 Roma Tomatoes
- 2 tbsp Chopped Onion
- 1 tsp. Sea Salt
- 1 tsp. Powdered onion
- 1 tsp. Oregano
- 2 tbsp. Agave
- 2 tbsp. Grape Seed Oil
- Basil (one Pinch)

Directions:

1. Create tiny x-shaped cuts on the ends of 5 plum tomatoes to remove the skin, then put them for 1 minute in boiling water.

2. Keep the tomatoes in ice-cold water for 30 seconds to enable quick peeling of the skin.

3. In your food processor or blender, combine the tomatoes and other ingredients for 30 seconds, or until smooth.

Alkaline Barbeque Sauce

This recipe will make about 8-10 oz. of barbecue sauce.

Ingredients

- 6 Tomatoes with Plum
- 2 tbsp. Agave
- 1/4 cup Sugar Date
- 1/4 cup White Onions, diced
- 2 tsp. Smoked Sea Salt
- 2 Tsp. Powdered onion
- 1/2 tsp. Ginger
- 1/4 tsp. Cayenne Powder
- 1/8 tsp. Cloves
- Mixer
- Hand blender

Directions

1. Combine all the ingredients to blend and blend until smooth, excluding date sugar.

2. Pour the combined ingredients and date sugar into a pan over medium-high heat and stir regularly until it boils.

3. Reduce heat to a simmer, then cover for 15 minutes with a plate, stirring periodically.

Dr. Sebi Diet

4. Using stick blender to smooth out the sauce.

5. Cook for 10 minutes over low heat or until the water evaporates off.

6. Let the sauce to cool and thicken further before serving.

7. Enjoy the Barbecue Alkaline sauce!

Guacamole

Ingredients

- 1 Orange Pepper
- 2 Roma Tomatoes
- 1 Jalapeños
- 1 Lime
- 4 Avocados
- 1 Red Onion
- Black Pepper (add as desired)
- Natural Sea Salt (add as desired)
- Himalayan Pink Sea Salt (add as desired)
- 2 Green Onions
- Extra Virgin Olive Oil (add as desired)

Directions

1. Cut the ingredients that require this after washing and then put it in a container.
2. Add extra virgin olive oil
3. Blend (as required)
4. Add diced tomatoes at the end (when mixed)

Onion Avocado Dip

Ingredients

- 3 medium-sized onions, chopped
- 1 avocado, chopped

Dr. Sebi Diet

- 8 plum or cherry tomatoes

- Juice of 1 medium-sized orange

- 1/2 teaspoon salt

- 1/2 teaspoon cayenne pepper

- 1 tablespoon fresh herbs

- 1 teaspoon olive oil (optional)

Direction

1. Pour everything in a food processor or blender and combine it to the texture needed.

2. Serve and chill.

Pairing suggestions

- Use over food instead of gravy

- Pour over salad

- General dip

Blend with small quantity orange juice to make it thicker in consistency and use in place of spread.

Note: Do not store for more than 1 day as it may spoil easily as tomatoes and avocados tend not to last long once used.

Marijuana Guacamole

Ingredients

- 3 avocados – peeled, pitted, and mashed

- 3 tablespoons chopped fresh cilantro

- 2 plum tomatoes, diced

- 2 teaspoons of crushed cannabis

Dr. Sebi Diet

- 1 lime, juiced

- 1 teaspoon salt

- 1 teaspoon of Cannabis oil

- 1 pinch ground cayenne pepper

- 1/2 cup diced onion

Directions

1. Mash the avocados, the lime juice, cannabis oil, and salt in a small cup. Mix together the onions, cilantro, cannabis, and tomatoes. Toss in the cayenne pepper.

2. For better taste, refrigerate 1 hour, or serve immediately.

Mango Papaya Seed Dressing

This recipe yields about 1/2 cup of dressing.

Ingredients

- 1 cup Mango
- 1/4 cup Grapeseed Oil
- 2 tbsp. Juice of lime
- 1 tsp. Papaya Seed
- 1 tsp. Agave
- 1 tsp. Basil
- 1 tsp. Powdered onion
- 1/4 tsp. sea Salt

Directions

1. Blend everything in a blender for about 1 minute, then it is ready to eat.

Note: The dressing stays in the refrigerator for around 2 days. You may season the dressing to your taste too.

Cucumber Dill Dressing

Dr. Sebi Diet

This recipe yields about 1/2 cup of dressing.

Ingredients

- 1 cup Cucumber
- 1/4 cup Avocado Oil
- 1 tablespoon. Juice of lime
- 2 tsp. Agave
- 1 tsp. Fresh Dill
- 1/2 tsp. Powdered onion

Directions

1. Blend everything in a blender for around 1 minute, then it is ready to eat.

Note: The dressing remains in the refrigerator for around 2 days. Bear in mind that fresh dill comes with a better flavor than dried dill. You may season the dressing to your taste too.

Red Ginger Dressing

This recipe yields about 1/2 cup of dressing.

Ingredients

- 2 Tomatoes plum, sliced
- 2 tbsp. Sesame seeds
- 1 tbsp. Onion
- 1 table spoon Agave
- 1 tbsp. Juice of lime
- 1 tsp. Ginger

Directions

1. Blend everything in a blender for around 1 minute, then it is ready to eat.

Dr. Sebi Diet

Note: The dressing remains in the refrigerator for around 2 days. Bear in mind that fresh dill comes with a better flavour than dried dill. You may season the dressing to your taste too.

Creamy Salad Dressing

Ingredients

- 4 tbs. almond butter
- 2 green onions
- 1/4 tsp. ground cumin
- 1/2 cup fresh lime juice
- 1/2 tsp. sweet basil
- 1/4 tsp. thyme
- 1 tsp. maple syrup
- 1/4 tsp. sea salt

Directions

1. Add all ingredients in a glass bottle and pour in 2 tablespoons of spring water
2. Shake thoroughly and enjoy

Cream of Kamut

Ingredients

- 4 cups of almond milk
- 2 cups of water
- 1 1/2 cup of kamut flour
- 1 1/2 tsp of vanilla extract
- 1 cup of maple crystals
- 1 tsp of cinnamon

Directions

1. Make like cream of rye.

Alkaline Electric Butter

This recipe will make about 14 oz. of butter.

Ingredients

- 3/4 cup of coconut oil
- 3/4 cup of grape seed oil
- 1/4 cup of spring water
- 1 tsp. Sea Moss Gel
- 1/2 tsp. sea salt

You may also try to create a herb butter by adding to the blend onion powder, basil, oregano, or other approved herbs by Dr. Sebi.

Directions

1. Stir the sea salt into the spring water at room temperature to dissolve.

2. Mix all ingredients together for 30 seconds with stick mixer.

3. Place in airtight container and refrigerate until solid. Store in freezer for around 20-25 minutes before placing in refrigerator for quicker output.

4. Enjoy the Alkaline Butter!

Brazil Nut Cheese

This recipe will make about 6 cups of cheese.

Ingredients

- 1 lb. Brazilian soaked nuts *
- 1/2 lime, juiced
- 2 tsp. Sea salt
- 1 tsp. Powdered onion
- 1/2 tsp. Cayenne

Dr. Sebi Diet

- 1 1/2 cup Cashew Milk, Hemp Milk, or any other Nut
- 1-1/2 cup spring water
- 2 tsp. Grapeseed oil
- blender or food processor
- Brazil nuts can be soaked overnight but if you don't have the time, soaking them for around 2 hours is perfect.

Directions

1. Combine all of the products, except the spring water, to your food processor or blender.

2. Blend ingredients together for 2 minutes, including just 1/2 cup of water.

3. Start adding 1/2 cup of water and mix until it achieves the perfect consistency.

4. Enjoy the Alkaline Brazilian Nut Cheese!

Dr. Sebi Diet

Conclusion

The diet approved by Dr. Sebi also known as Alfredo Bowman has permitted certain food items that are 100% vegan and are not processed or modified. Dr. Sebi is not a professional or does not hold any degree but he claims himself to be a self-taught herbalist. However following this diet can help prevent the diseases such as heart diseases, diabetes, kidney disorder or liver diseases. This diet can also be used to reduce weight and reverse or prevent the already mentioned health problems. Detoxification and cleansing has several health benefits even if it has few disadvantages. Few of the advantages of this are, it keeps you healthy and physically fit, boosts immunity, improve the focus of the person. Other than that there are also natural methods of detoxification such as dry brushing, cupping, souping, exercising etc. By adapting this diet, one can have several health benefits that are shinier hair, healthy and clear skin, improved immunity and overall optimal health. Recipes given in this book provides the individual with variety and versatility who is looking forward to follow the diet approved by Dr. Sebi. There are lot of combinations for the approved items that can be achieved and enjoyed.

References

10 Important Benefits of Detoxing Your Body – USA TODAY Classifieds. Retrieved from https://classifieds.usatoday.com/blog/business/10-important-benefits-detoxing-body/

5 Soups Recipes (Dr Sebi Approved Ingredients) - ital is vital. Retrieved from https://italisvital.info/5-soups-recipes-dr-sebi-approved-ingredients/

Dr Sebi Food List: The Best Electric and Alkaline Foods to Eat. Retrieved from https://www.blackhealthwealth.com/dr-sebi-food-list/

Dr Sebi's Herb List - ital is vital. Retrieved from https://italisvital.info/dr-sebis-herb-list/

Dr. Sebi diet review: Method, evidence, benefits, and risks. Retrieved from https://www.medicalnewstoday.com/articles/327399#who-is-dr-sebi

Everything to Know About the Dr. Sebi Diet. Retrieved from https://www.goodhousekeeping.com/health/diet-nutrition/a31290735/dr-sebi-diet-review/

Fatty Lever- Diseases and Ways to Detox. Retrieved from https://medium.com/@rawsomehealthy/fatty-lever-diseases-and-ways-to-detox-1921d27a0cd0

Full Body Detox: 9 Ways to Rejuvenate Your Body. Retrieved from https://www.healthline.com/nutrition/how-to-detox-your-body#section11

How to Detox for Digestive Issues. Retrieved from https://elevays.com/detox-for-digestive-issues/

CPSIA information can be obtained
at www.ICGtesting.com
Printed in the USA
BVHW012127200921
617169BV00009B/220